COMPLETE GU

THE NEW
GLUCOSE
revolution

**PROF JENNIE BRAND-MILLER
KAYE FOSTER-POWELL
DR SUSANNA HOLT**

HODDER

Other books in the New Glucose Revolution Series

The New Glucose Revolution
The New Glucose Revolution Life Plan
The New Glucose Revolution Childhood Diabetes
The New Glucose Revolution Healthy Kids
The New Glucose Revolution Heart Health
The New Glucose Revolution Losing Weight
The New Glucose Revolution Peak Performance
The New Glucose Revolution People with Diabetes
The New Glucose Revolution Sugar and Energy

A Hodder Book

Published in Australia and New Zealand in 2003
by Hodder Headline Australia Pty Limited
(A member of the Hodder Headline Group)
Level 22, 201 Kent Street, Sydney NSW 2000
Website: www.hha.com.au

Reprinted 2003 (four times)

The GI logo is a trademark of the University of Sydney in Australia and other
countries. A food product carrying this logo is nutritious and has been tested for
its GI by an accredited laboratory.

National Library of Australia
Cataloguing-in-Publication data

Brand Miller, Jennie, 1952- .
  The new glucose revolution : complete guide to GI values.

  ISBN 0 7336 1667 4.

  1. Dietetics. 2. Glycemic index. 3. Carbohydrates.
  4. Food – Carbohydrate content. I. Foster-Powell, Kaye.
  II. Holt, Susanna. III. Title.

613.283

Cover by Greendot design
Typesetting by Bookhouse, Sydney
Printed in Australia by Griffin Press, Adelaide

CONTENTS

Introduction   1

Understanding the glycemic index   5

Let's talk glycemic load   8

Your daily food choices   12

A to Z GI values   17

Food category GI values   50

Low to high GI values   109

INTRODUCTION

The GI values are the key to unlocking the enormous health benefits of *The New Glucose Revolution*.

People with diabetes, heart disease, the metabolic syndrome (Syndrome X) or people who are overweight will gain the most from putting *The New Glucose Revolution* approach into practice. But it's also for those who want to do the best they can to prevent those problems in the first place, and improve their overall health. In short, *The New Glucose Revolution* is for everybody.

With that in mind, we've put together this handy companion book full of GI values to help you put the GI into practice. There are three listings in this book:

- an A–Z list of individual foods for easy reference;
- a comprehensive list of foods and food categories for in-depth knowledge;
- and a simple food category list in GI value order for quick comparisons.

You can use the different listings to:

- find the GI of your favourite food
- compare foods within the same category (for instance, two types of bread) to see which is lower
- improve your diet by finding low GI substitutes for high GI foods
- find the lowest GI value within a food group easily
- compare the GI values of food groups
- put together a low GI meal
- shop for low GI foods
- check the GI value of products

If you can't find a GI value for a food you eat on many occasions, please write to the manufacturer and encourage them to have the GI of the food tested by an accredited laboratory such as Sydney University's Glycemic Index Research Service (SUGiRS). In the meantime, use a similar food as a substitute.

When you're grocery shopping, look out for those foods with the GI symbol. The GI symbol (pictured below) flags healthy foods that have been properly GI tested and includes their GI value on the packing. You might encourage companies to join the GI symbol program (see our website for more information www.glycemicindex.com).

The GI values in this book are correct at the time of publication. However, the formulation of commercial foods can change and the GI may be altered. You can rely on those foods showing the GI symbol. You will find revised and new data on our webpage www.glycemicindex.com.

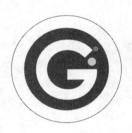

UNDERSTANDING THE GLYCEMIC INDEX

Our research on the GI began in the 1980s when health authorities all over the world began to stress the importance of high carbohydrate diets. Until then dietary fat had grabbed all the public and scientific attention (and to some extent this is still true). But low fat diets are by their very nature *automatically* high in carbohydrate. Nutrition scientists started asking questions—are all carbohydrates the same, are all starches good for health, are all sugars bad? In particular, they began studies on the effects of carbohydrates on blood glucose levels. They wanted to know which carbohydrate foods were associated with the least fluctuation in blood glucose levels and the best overall health, including a reduced risk of diabetes and heart disease.

As we explain in our bestselling book, *The New Glucose Revolution*, the glycemic index:

- is a scientifically proven measure of the effect carbohydrates have on blood glucose levels;
- helps you choose the right amount and type of carbohydrate for your health and wellbeing;
- provides an easy and effective way to eat a healthy diet and control fluctuations in blood glucose.

What is the GI

The GI is a physiologically based measure of carbohydrate quality—a comparison of carbohydrates (gram for gram) based on their immediate effects on blood glucose levels.

- Carbohydrates that break down quickly during digestion have high GI values. Their blood glucose response is fast and high.
- Carbohydrates that break down slowly, releasing glucose gradually into the bloodstream, have a low GI.

The rate of carbohydrate digestion has important implications for everybody. For most people, the foods with a low GI have advantages over those with high GI. This is especially true for people with diabetes or trying to control their weight.

A knowledge and appreciation of the GI will help you choose the right amount of carbohydrate and the right sort of carbohydrate for your lifestyle and well-being. We know from our own experience and letters from our readers that understanding the GI of foods makes an enormous difference to people's lives. For some it means a new lease of life.

For more detailed information about the GI, it effects and benefits, you should consult our other books, *The New Glucose Revolution* and *The New Glucose Revolution Life Plan*. These books also provide practical advice and tips about changing to low GI diets, improving your overall diet, foods to stock and buy, and delicious recipes to try.

LET'S TALK GLYCEMIC LOAD

As well as the GI values, the lists in this book include the glycemic load (GL) value of average-sized portions of the foods to ensure you have all the information you need to choose foods which will improve your overall health.

Glycemic load is the product of the GI and carbohydrate per serve of food. When we eat a meal containing carbohydrate, the blood glucose rises and falls. The extent to which it rises and remains high is critically important to health and depends on two things: the *amount* of a carbohydrate in the meal and the *nature* (GI) of that carbohydrate. Both are equally important determinants of changes in blood glucose levels.

Researchers at Harvard University came up with a way of combining and describing these two factors with the term 'glycemic load'. It provides a measure of the degree of glycemia and insulin demand produced by a normal serving of the food. GI values are measured for fixed portions of foods containing a certain amount of carbohydrate, usually 50 grams. However, as people eat different sized portions of the same foods, we can work out the extent to which a certain portion of food will raise the blood glucose level by calculating a glycemic load value for that amount of food.

Glycemic load is calculated simply by mulitplying the GI of a food by the amount of carbohydrate in that serving and dividing by 100.

$$\text{Glycemic load} = (\text{GI} \times \text{carbohydrate per serving}) \div 100$$

For example, an apple has a GI of 40 and contains 15 grams of carbohydrate per serve. Its glycemic load is $(40 \times 15) \div 100 = 6$. A potato has a GI of 90 and 20 grams of carbohydrate per serve. It has a glycemic load of $(90 \times 20) \div 100 = 18$. This means one potato will raise your blood glucose level higher than one apple.

The glycemic load is greatest for those foods which provide the most high GI carbohydrate, particularly those we tend to eat in large quantities. Compare the glycemic load of the following foods to see how the serving size as well as the GI are significant in determining the glycemic response:

Rice—1 cup of boiled white rice (150 g) contains 43 g carbohydrate and has a GI of 83. The glycemic load is $(83 \times 43) \div 100 = 36$.

Spaghetti—1 serve (150 g) of cooked spaghetti contains 48 g carbohydrate and has a GI of 44. The glycemic load is $(44 \times 48) \div 100 = 21$.

Some nutritionists have argued that the glycemic load is an improvement on the GI because it provides an estimate of both quantity and quality of carbohydrate (the GI gives us just quality) in a diet. In large scale studies from Harvard University, however, the risk of disease was predicted by both the GI of the overall diet as well as the glycemic load. The use of the glycemic load strengthened the relationship, suggesting that the more frequent the consumption of high carbohydrate, high GI foods, the more adverse the health outcome. Carbohydrate by itself has no effect, ie there was no benefit of low carbohydrate intake over high carbohydrate intake, or vice versa.

Low GL = 10 or less
Intermediate GL = 11–19
High GL = 20 or more

Don't make the mistake of using GL alone. If you do, you might find yourself eating a diet with very little carbohydrate but a lot of fat, especially saturated fat, and excessive amounts of protein. Use the glycemic index to compare foods of similar nature (eg bread with bread) and use the glycemic load when comparing foods with a high GI but low carbohydrate content per serve (eg pumpkin).

Remember that the GL values listed are for the specified (nominal) portion size listed. If you eat a different portion size (ie weight), then you will need to calculate another GL value. First find out the GI of your food, then the weight of your portion and then work out the available carbohydrate content of this weight (this value is listed beside the GL). For example, the GI of pumpkin is 75, the nominal serve size is 80 grams and the available carbohydrate is 4 grams. So the current GL is $(75 \times 4) \div 100 = 3$. If, however, you were eating twice the nominal size (160 grams, in this instance) you would need to double the available carbohydrate (8 grams, in this example) and the GL for your larger serve of pumpkin would be: $(75 \times 8) \div 100 = 6$.

YOUR DAILY FOOD CHOICES

To guide your daily food choices we've created two GI food pyramids, one for moderate carbohydrate eaters and one for high carbohydrate eaters. The recommended servings of each food group are shown on each pyramid. If you are a big bread and cereal eater, the GI pyramid for high carbohydrate eaters will suit you best. Either way, the serving information on page 15 applies to both pyramids.

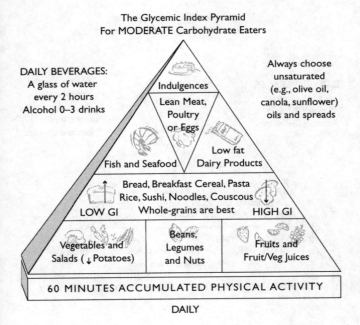

The Glycemic Index Pyramid
For MODERATE Carbohydrate Eaters

For moderate carbohydrate eaters:

Indulgences: 1–2 servings

Fish and seafood / Lean meat, poultry and eggs: 2–3 servings

Low fat dairy products: 2–3 servings

Bread, breakfast cereals, grains: 4–6 servings

Vegetables and salads: 4–6 servings

Beans, legumes and nuts: 1–2 serving

Fruits and juices: 2–3 servings

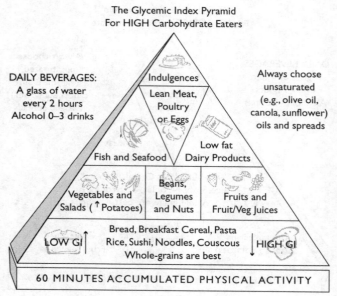

The Glycemic Index Pyramid
For HIGH Carbohydrate Eaters

DAILY BEVERAGES:
A glass of water
every 2 hours
Alcohol 0–3 drinks

Indulgences

Lean Meat,
Poultry
or Eggs

Always choose
unsaturated
(e.g., olive oil,
canola, sunflower)
oils and spreads

Fish and Seafood

Low fat
Dairy Products

Vegetables and
Salads (↑ Potatoes)

Beans,
Legumes
and Nuts

Fruits and
Fruit/Veg Juices

LOW GI ↑

Bread, Breakfast Cereal, Pasta
Rice, Sushi, Noodles, Couscous
Whole-grains are best

↓ HIGH GI

60 MINUTES ACCUMULATED PHYSICAL ACTIVITY

DAILY

For high carbohydrate eaters:

Indulgences: 1–2 servings

Fish and seafood / Lean meat, poultry and eggs: 2–3 servings

Low fat dairy products: 2–3 servings

Bread, breakfast cereals, grains etc: 6–8 servings

Vegetables and salads: 4–6 servings

Beans, legumes and nuts: 1 serving

Fruits and juices: 3–4 servings

Serving information

The following answers the question of how much is a serve. The one set serves both pyramids.

INDULGENCES:

1 Tbsp (20 g) butter, margarine, oil
2 Tbsp (40 g) cream, mayonnaise
25 g chocolate
1 small slice (40 g) cake
1 small packet (30 g) potato crisps
2 standard alcoholic drinks alcohol

FISH AND SEAFOOD / LEAN MEAT, POULTRY AND EGGS:

80–120 g cooked fish
60–90 g cooked lean meat or poultry
1 egg

LOW FAT DAIRY PRODUCTS:

1 cup (250 ml) low fat milk or yoghurt
40 g reduced fat cheese

BREAD, BREAKFAST CEREALS, GRAINS ETC:

1 slice bread
30 g cereal
½ cup cooked rice, pasta or noodles

VEGETABLES & SALADS:
½ cup cooked vegetables
1 cup raw, salad vegetables

BEANS, LEGUMES AND NUTS:
1 cup cooked dried beans, peas or lentils
30 g nuts

FRUITS AND JUICES:
1 medium piece of fruit
1 cup of small fruit pieces
½ cup juice

A TO Z
GI VALUES

This is the place to go when you want to locate the GI value of a popular food quickly. Here foods are listed alphabetically—both on an individual basis and within their specific food category. For example, you will find Bürgen breads under both Breads and Bürgen. Food category entries include: biscuits, breads, breakfast cereal bars, breakfast cereals, cereal grains, crackers, dairy products, fruit, fruit juices, legumes, meat, pasta and noodles, potato, rice, snack foods, soft drinks, soups, sports drinks, sugars and honey, and vegetables.

We have also included some foods under their well-known brand or company names as well, for example Norco ice-cream appears as both 'Ice-cream (Norco)' and 'Norco Ice-cream'.

This a condensed listing of the GI values: we have given the average GI values for some foods. The average value may be calculated from the results of 10 separate studies of that food worldwide or only 2 to 4 studies. In a few instances, Australian data are different to the rest of the world and we show our data rather than the average. The food category listings on pages 48–104 are more comprehensive, showing the different studies and worldwide results.

In this listing you'll find not only the GI but the glycemic load (GL = carbohydrate content × GI/100). The glycemic load has been calculated using a 'nominal' serving size and the carbohydrate content of that serve, both of which are also listed. In this way, you can choose foods with either a low GI and/or a low GL. If your favourite food is both high GI and high GL, try to cut down the serving size or dilute the GL by teaming it with a very low GI food (eg rice and lentils).

We've also included some foods that contain very little carbohydrate and have therefore been automatically omitted from previous editions. However, so many people ask us for their GI, we decided the best thing was to include them and show their GI as [0]. Many vegetables such as avocadoes and broccoli, and protein-rich foods such as eggs, chicken, cheese and tuna are among the low or no carbohydrate category. Most alcoholic beverages are also low in carbohydrate. Beer has approximately 10 grams per middy, but its GI is unknown.

FOOD	GI	NOMINAL SERVE SIZE	AVAILABLE CARB PER SERVE	GL PER SERVE
All-Bran™, breakfast cereal	30	30 g	15	4
All-Bran Fruit 'n' Oats™, breakfast cereal	39	30 g	17	7
All-Bran Soy 'n' Fibre™, breakfast cereal	33	30 g	14	4
Angel food cake, 1 slice	67	50 g	29	19
Apple, raw, 1 medium	38*	120 g	15	6
Apple, dried	29	60 g	34	10
Apple juice, pure, unsweetened	40	250 ml	28	11
Apple muffin	44	60 g	29	13
Apple, oat and sultana muffin (from packet mix)	54	50 g	26	14
Apricots, raw, 3 medium	57	168 g	13	7
Apricots, canned in light syrup	64	120 g	19	12
Apricots, dried	30	60 g	27	8
Apricot, coconut and honey muffin (from mix)	60	50 g	26	16
Arborio, risotto rice, white, boiled	69	150 g	43	29
Bagel, white	72	70 g	35	25
Baked beans, canned in tomato sauce	48*	150 g	17	8
Banana, raw, 1 large	52*	120 g	26	13
Banana cake, 1 slice	47	80 g	38	18
Banana, oat and honey muffin (from packet mix)	65	50 g	26	17
Barley, pearled, boiled	25*	150 g	32	8
Basmati rice, white, boiled, 1 cup	58	150 g	42	24
Beef	[0]	120 g	0	0
Beer	[0]	250 ml	10 g	0
Beetroot, canned	64	80 g	7	5
Bengal gram dhal, chickpea	11	150 g	36	4
Biscuits Digestives	59*	25 g	16	10

* Average

19

FOOD	GI	NOMINAL SERVE SIZE	AVAILABLE CARB PER SERVE	GL PER SERVE
Highland Oatmeal™	55	25 g	18	10
Milk Arrowroot™	69	25 g	18	12
Morning Coffee™	79	25 g	19	15
Shortbread	64	25 g	16	10
Shredded Wheatmeal™	62	25 g	18	11
Snack Right™ Fruit Slice	48	25 g	19	9
Black bean soup	64	250 ml	27	17
Black beans, boiled	30	150 g	25	5
Blackbread (Riga)	76	30 g	13	10
Blackeyed beans, soaked, boiled	42	150 g	29	12
Blueberry muffin	59	57 g	29	17
Bran Flakes™, breakfast cereal	74	30 g	18	13
Bran muffin	60	57 g	24	15
Breads				
Bagel, white	72	70 g	35	25
Baguette, white	95	30 g	15	15
Barley flour bread	67	30 g	13	9
Blackbread (Riga)	76	30 g	13	10
Bürgen™ Oatbran and Honey	49	40 g	13	7
Bürgen™ Rye	51	40 g	13	7
Bürgen® Soy-Lin	36	30 g	9	3
Continental fruit loaf	47	30 g	15	7
Fruit and Spice Loaf (Buttercup)	54	30 g	15	8
Gluten-free multigrain bread	79	30 g	13	10
Hamburger bun, white	61	30 g	15	9
Helga's™ Classic Seed Loaf	68	30 g	14	9
Helga's™ traditional wholemeal bread	70	30 g	13	9
Hyfibre, white	70	67 g	27	19
Holsom's, sunflower and poppyseed	61	74 g	30	18

* Average

FOOD	GI	NOMINAL SERVE SIZE	AVAILABLE CARB PER SERVE	GL PER SERVE
Holsom's wholemeal and rye	63	74 g	28	18
Kaiser rolls	73	30 g	16	12
Lebanese bread, white	75	30 g	16	12
Melba toast	70	30 g	23	16
Multigrain Spelt wheat loaf	54	30 g	15	8
Multigrain (Tip Top)	65	30 g	28	18
9-Grain Multi-Grain (Tip-Top)	43	30 g	14	6
Pain au lait	63	60 g	32	20
Performax™ (Country Life)	38	30 g	13	5
Pita bread	57	30 g	17	10
Ploughman's™ Wholegrain	47	30 g	14	7
Ploughman's™ Wholemeal	64	30 g	13	9
Rice bread, high-amylose Doongara rice	61	30 g	12	7
Rice bread, low-amylose Calrose rice	72	30 g	12	8
Roggenbrot (Vogel's)	59	30 g	14	8
Schinkenbrot (Riga)	86	30 g	14	12
Sourdough rye	53*	30 g	12	6
Sourdough wheat	54	30 g	14	8
Spelt multigrain bread	54	30 g	12	7
Sunflower and barley bread (Riga)	57	30 g	11	6
Vogel's Honey & Oats	55	30 g	14	7
White bread	70	30 g	14	10
Wholemeal bread	77	30 g	12	9
Wholemeal rye bread	58*	30 g	14	8
Wonderwhite™ (Buttercup)	80	30 g	14	11
Breakfast cereal bars				
Crunchy Nut Cornflakes™ bar	72	30 g	26	19
Fibre Plus™ bar	78	30 g	23	18

* Average

21

FOOD	GI	NOMINAL SERVE SIZE	AVAILABLE CARB PER SERVE	GL PER SERVE
Fruity-Bix™ bar, fruit and nut	56	30 g	19	10
Fruity-Bix™ bar, wild berry	51	30 g	19	9
K-Time Just Right™ bar	72	30 g	24	17
K-Time Strawberry Crunch™ bar	77	30 g	25	19
Rice Bubble Treat™ bar	63	30 g	24	15
Sustain™ bar	57	30 g	25	14
Breakfast cereals				
All-Bran™	30	30 g	15	5
All-Bran Fruit 'n' Oats™	39	30 g	17	7
All-Bran Soy 'n' Fibre™	33	30 g	14	4
Bran Flakes™	74	30 g	18	13
Coco Pops™	77	30 g	26	20
Cornflakes™	77	30 g	25	20
Cornflakes, Crunchy Nut™	72	30 g	24	17
Corn Pops™	80	30 g	26	21
Froot Loops™	69	30 g	26	18
Frosties™	55	30 g	26	15
Golden Wheats™	71	30 g	23	16
Good Start™, muesli wheat biscuits	68	30 g	20	14
Guardian™	37	30 g	12	5
Healthwise™ for bowel health	66	30 g	18	12
Healthwise™ for heart health	48	30 g	19	9
Hi-Bran Weet-Bix™	61	30 g	17	10
Hi-Bran Weet-Bix™ with soy and linseed	57	30 g	16	9
Hyfibre, white sandwich bread	70	67 g	27	19
Holsom's sunflower and poppyseed bread	61	74 g	30	18

* Average

FOOD	GI	NOMINAL SERVE SIZE	AVAILABLE CARB PER SERVE	GL PER SERVE
Holsom's wholemeal and rye bread	63	74 g	28	18
Honey Goldies™	72	30 g	21	15
Honey Rice Bubbles™	77	30 g	27	20
Honey Smacks™	71	30 g	23	16
Just Right™	60	30 g	22	13
Just Right Just Grains™	62	30 g	23	14
Komplete™	48	30 g	21	10
Lite-Bix™, no added sugar	70	30 g	20	14
Mini Wheats™, whole wheat	58	30 g	21	12
Mini Wheats™, blackcurrant	72	30 g	21	15
Muesli, gluten-free	39	30 g	19	7
Muesli, Natural	48*	30 g	18	8
Muesli, toasted (Purina)	43	30 g	17	7
Nutrigrain™	66	30 g	15	10
Oat 'n' Honey Bake™	77	30 g	17	13
Oat bran Weet-Bix™	57	30 g	20	11
Porridge, made from whole rolled oats	55*	250 g	21	11
Porridge, traditional oats	51	250 g	21	11
Porridge, instant	66*	250 g	26	17
Pop Tarts™, chocolate	70	50 g	36	25
Puffed Wheat	80	30 g	21	17
Rice Bran, extruded (Rice Growers)	19	30 g	14	3
Rice Bubbles™	87	30 g	26	22
Shredded Wheat	75	30 g	20	15
Soy Tasty™	60	30 g	20	12
Soytana™ (Vogel's)	49	45 g	25	12
Special K™	54	30 g	21	11
Sultana Bran™	73	30 g	19	14

* Average

FOOD	GI	NOMINAL SERVE SIZE	AVAILABLE CARB PER SERVE	GL PER SERVE
Sultana Goldies™	65	30 g	21	13
Sustain™	68	30 g	22	15
Ultra-bran™, soy and linseed	41	30 g	13	5
Vita-Brits™	68	30 g	20	13
Wheat-bites™	72	30 g	25	18
Weet-Bix™	69	30 g	17	12
Whole wheat Goldies™	70	30 g	20	14
Breton™ wheat crackers	67	25 g	14	10
Broad beans	79	80 g	11	9
Broken rice, white, cooked in rice cooker	86	150 g	43	37
Buckwheat, boiled	54*	150 g	30	16
Buckwheat, pancakes, gluten-free, made from packet mix	102	77 g	22	22
Bulghur, boiled 20 min	48*	150 g	26	12
Bun, hamburger	61	30 g	15	9
Bürgen® Oat Bran & Honey	49	40 g	13	7
Bürgen® Soy-Lin, kibbled soy (8%) and linseed (8%) loaf	36	30 g	9	3
Bürgen® Fruit Loaf	44	30 g	13	6
Bürgen® Mixed Grain	49*	30 g	11	6
Burger Rings™, barbeque-flavoured	90	50 g	31	28
Butter beans, dried, boiled	31*	150 g	20	6
Calrose rice, white, medium grain, boiled	83	150 g	42	35
Capellini pasta, boiled	45	180 g	45	20
Capsicum	[0]	80 g	0	0
Carrots, peeled, boiled	41*	80 g	5	2
Cereal grains				
Arborio, risotto rice, boiled	69	150 g	53	36
Barley, rolled, dry	66	50 g	38	25

* Average

FOOD	GI	NOMINAL SERVE SIZE	AVAILABLE CARB PER SERVE	GL PER SERVE
Basmati rice, boiled, white (Mahatma, Australia)	58	150 g	38	22
Buckwheat, boiled	54	150 g	30	16
Calrose rice, brown, boiled	87	150 g	38	33
Calrose rice, white, medium grain, boiled	83	150 g	43	36
Cornmeal, boiled	69	150 g	13	9
Corn, sweet	48	150 g	30	14
Couscous	65	150 g	33	21
Cracked wheat (bulghur), cooked	48*	150 g	26	12
Doongara rice, brown, boiled	66	150 g	37	24
Doongara rice, white	56	150 g	39	22
Instant rice, white, cooked 6 min	87	150 g	42	36
Instant Doongara rice, white	94	150 g	42	35
Koshikari (Japanese) white rice, boiled	48	150 g	42	20
Jasmine rice	109	150 g	42	46
Long grain rice, boiled	56	150 g	41	23
Parboiled, Doongara rice, boiled	50	150 g	39	19
Parboiled rice, Sungold	87	150 g	39	34
Pearl Barley, boiled	25	150 g	32	8
Pelde rice, brown, boiled	76	150 g	38	29
Pelde rice, white	93	150 g	43	40
Rice, brown, boiled	55	150 g	33	18
Rice, boiled, white	56	150 g	42	23
Rye, whole kernels, cooked	34	50 g	38	13
Semolina, cooked	55	150 g	11	6
Sunbrown rice, Quick™, boiled	80	150 g	38	31
Sungold rice, Pelde, parboiled	87	150 g	43	37
Wheat, whole kernels, cooked	41	50 g	34	14
Wheat, quick-cooking kernels	54	150 g	47	25

* Average

FOOD	GI	NOMINAL SERVE SIZE	AVAILABLE CARB PER SERVE	GL PER SERVE
Cheese	[0]	120 g	0	0
Cherries, raw	22	120 g	12	3
Chickpeas, canned in brine	42	150 g	22	9
Chickpeas, dried, boiled	28*	150 g	24	7
Chicken nuggets, frozen, reheated in microwave oven 5 min	46	100 g	16	7
Chocolate, plain, milk	43*	50 g	28	12
Chocolate, white, Milky Bar®	44	50 g	29	13
Chocolate butterscotch muffins, made from packet mix	53	50 g	28	15
Chocolate cake made from packet mix with chocolate frosting	38	111 g	52	20
Chocolate mousse, 2% fat	31	50 g	11	3
Chocolate pudding, instant made from packet with whole milk	47	100 g	16	7
Coca Cola®, soft drink	53	250 ml	26	14
Coco Pops™	77	30 g	26	20
Condensed milk, sweetened, full-fat	61	50 ml	28	17
Cordial, orange, reconstituted	66	250 ml	20	13
Corn chips, plain, salted	42	50 g	25	11
Cornflakes™, breakfast cereal	77	30 g	25	20
Cornflakes Crunchy Nut™, breakfast cereal	72	30 g	24	17
Cornmeal, boiled in salted water 2 min	68	150 g	13	9
Corn pasta, gluten-free, boiled	78	180 g	42	32
Corn Pops™, breakfast cereal	80	30 g	26	21
Corn Thins, puffed corn cakes, gluten-free	87	25 g	20	18
Couscous, boiled 5 min	65*	150 g	33	21
Crackers				
Breton wheat crackers	67	25 g	14	10

* Average

FOOD	GI	NOMINAL SERVE SIZE	AVAILABLE CARB PER SERVE	GL PER SERVE
Jatz™, plain salted crackers	55	25 g	17	10
Kavli™ Norwegian Crispbread	71	25 g	16	12
Puffed Crispbread	81	25 g	19	15
Puffed rice cakes	82	25 g	21	17
Rye crispbread	64	25 g	16	11
Sao™, plain square crackers	70	25 g	17	12
Vita-wheat™, original, crispbread	55	25 g	19	10
Water cracker	78	25 g	18	14
Cranberry juice cocktail	52	250 ml	31	16
Crispix™, breakfast cereal	87	30 g	25	22
Croissant	67	57 g	26	17
Crumpet, white	69	50 g	19	13
Crunchy Nut Cornflakes™ bar	72	30 g	26	19
Crunchy Nut™ Cornflakes	72	30 g	24	17
Cupcake, strawberry-iced	73	38 g	26	19
Custard, home made from milk, (wheat starch), and sugar	43	100 ml	17	7
Custard, prepared from powder with whole milk, No Bake™ (Nestlé)	35	100 ml	17	6
Custard, TRIM™, reduced-fat	37	100 ml	15	6
Custard apple, raw, flesh only	54	120 g	19	10
Dairy products				
Custard	38*	100 ml	16	6
Ice-cream, reduced	61	50 g	13	8
Peter's Light Ice-cream, vanilla, low-fat	50	50 g	6	3
Ice-cream, vanilla Prestige Light™ (Norco, Australia)	47	50 g	10	5
Ice-cream, Prestige Light™ traditional toffee (Norco, Australia)	37	50 g	14	5

* Average

FOOD	GI	NOMINAL SERVE SIZE	AVAILABLE CARB PER SERVE	GL PER SERVE
Ice-cream, Prestige™, golden macadamia (Norco, Australia)	37	50 g	9	3
Ice-cream, Premium Ultra chocolate, 15% fat (Sara Lee, Australia)	37	50 g	9	4
Ice-cream, French vanilla, 16% fat (Sara Lee, Australia)	38	50 g	9	3
Milk, full-fat, fresh	31	250 ml	12	4
Milk, low fat, chocolate, no added sugar	24	250 ml	15	3
Milk, chocolate, sugar-sweetened	43	50 ml	28	12
Mousse, reduced fat, from mix	34*	50 g	10	4
Peter's light & creamy™ vanilla ice-cream	44	50 g	13	6
Yoghurt, low fat, fruit, aspartame, Ski™	14	200 ml	13	2
Low fat, fruit, sugar, Ski™	33	200 ml	31	10
Yoghurt, no-fat, French vanilla, Vaalia, with sugar	40	150 ml	27	10
Yoghurt, no-fat, Mango, Vaalia, with sugar	39	150 ml	25	10
Yoghurt, no-fat, Wildberry, Vaalia, with sugar	38	150 ml	22	8
Yoghurt, no-fat, Strawberry, Vaalia, with sugar	38	150 ml	22	8
Yoghurt drink, Reduced-fat Vaalia™, passionfruit	38	200 ml	29	11
Dark rye, Blackbread (Riga)	76	30 g	13	10
Dark rye, Schinkenbrot (Riga)	86	30 g	14	12
Dates, dried	103	60 g	40	42
Desiree potato, peeled, boiled 35 min	101	150 g	17	17
Dietworks™ Hazelnut & Apricot bar	42	50 g	22	9

* Average

FOOD	GI	NOMINAL SERVE SIZE	AVAILABLE CARB PER SERVE	GL PER SERVE
Digestives plain, 2 biscuits	59*	25 g	16	10
Doongara, rice, white, boiled	56*	150 g	42	24
Egg Custard, prepared from powdered mix with whole milk, no bake	35	100 ml	17	6
Eggs	[0]	120 g	0	0
Ensure™, vanilla drink	48	250 ml	34	16
Ensure™ bar, chocolate fudge brownie	43	38 g	20	8
Ensure Plus™, vanilla drink	40	237 ml	40	19
Ensure Pudding™, old-fashioned vanilla	36	113 g	26	9
Fanta®, orange soft drink	68	250 ml	34	23
Fettuccine, egg, cooked	32	180 g	46	15
Figs, dried, tenderised	61	60 g	26	16
Fish	[0]	120 g	0	0
Fish fillet, crumbed (Maggi)	43	85 g	16	7
Fish Fingers	38	100 g	19	7
French baguette, white, plain	95	30 g	15	15
French fries, frozen, reheated in microwave	75	150 g	29	22
French vanilla ice-cream, premium, 16% fat (Sara Lee)	38	50 g	9	3
Froot Loops™, breakfast cereal	69	30 g	26	18
Frosties™, sugar-coated Cornflakes	55	30 g	26	15
Fructose, pure	19*	10 g	10	2
Vanilla cake made from packet mix with vanilla frosting	42	111 g	58	24
Fruit				
Apple	38*	120 g	15	6
Apple, dried	29	60 g	34	10
Apricots, dried	31*	60 g	28	9

* Average

FOOD	GI	NOMINAL SERVE SIZE	AVAILABLE CARB PER SERVE	GL PER SERVE
Banana	52*	120 g	26	13
Cherries	22	120 g	12	3
Dates, dried	103	60 g	40	42
Figs, dried	61	60 g	26	16
Grapefruit	25	120 g	11	3
Grapes, raw	46*	120 g	18	8
Grapes, black	59	120 g	18	11
Kiwi fruit	53*	120 g	12	6
Lychee, canned in syrup, drained	79	120 g	20	16
Mango	51*	120 g	17	8
Oranges	42*	120 g	11	5
Paw paw	59*	120 g	8	5
Peach	42*	120 g	11	5
Peach, canned in natural juice	38	120 g	11	4
Pears	38*	120 g	11	4
Pear halves, canned in reduced-sugar syrup, (SPC Lite)	25	120 g	14	4
Pear halves, canned in natural juice (SPC)	43	120 g	13	5
Pineapple, raw	59*	120 g	13	7
Plum, raw	39*	120 g	12	5
Prunes, pitted (Sunsweet)	29	60 g	33	10
Raisins	64	60 g	44	28
Rockmelon	65	120 g	6	4
Strawberries	40	120 g	3	1
Sultanas	56	60 g	45	25
Watermelon, raw	72	120 g	6	4
Fruit cocktail, canned	55	120 g	16	9
Fruit Fingers, Heinz Kidz™, banana	61	30 g	20	12
Fruit Juices				
Apple juice, unsweetened	40	250 ml	29	12

* Average

FOOD	GI	NOMINAL SERVE SIZE	AVAILABLE CARB PER SERVE	GL PER SERVE
Apple juice, pure, clear (Wild About Fruit, Australia)	44	250 ml	30	13
Apple juice, pure, cloudy (Wild About Fruit, Australia)	37	250 ml	28	10
Carrot juice, fresh	43	250 ml	23	10
Cranberry juice cocktail	52	250 ml	31	16
Grapefruit juice, unsweetened	48	250 ml	22	11
Orange juice, unsweetened	50*	250 ml	19	9
Pineapple juice, unsweetened	46	250 ml	34	16
Tomato juice, canned, no added sugar	38	250 ml	9	4
Fruit loaf, Bürgen™	44	30 g	13	6
Fruit Loaf, dense continental style wheat bread with dried fruit	47	30 g	15	7
Fruit and Spice Loaf, thick sliced	54	30 g	15	8
Gatorade® sports drink	78	250 ml	15	12
Glucodin™ glucose tablets	102	10 g	10	10
Gluten-free white bread, sliced	80	30 g	15	12
Gluten-free multigrain bread	79	30 g	13	10
Gluten-free muesli, with 1.5% fat milk	39	30 g	19	7
Gluten-free corn pasta	78	180 g	42	32
Gluten-free rice and maize pasta	76	180 g	49	37
Gluten-free split pea and soy pasta shells	29	180 g	31	9
Gluten-free spaghetti, rice and split pea, canned in tomato sauce	68	220 g	27	19
Glutinous rice, white, cooked in rice cooker	98	150 g	32	31
Gnocchi, cooked (Latina)	68	180 g	48	33
Golden Wheats™, breakfast cereal	71	30 g	23	16
Grapefruit, raw	25	120 g	11	3
Grapefruit juice, unsweetened	48	250 ml	20	9

* Average

FOOD	GI	NOMINAL SERVE SIZE	AVAILABLE CARB PER SERVE	GL PER SERVE
Grapes, green	46*	120 g	18	8
Green pea soup, canned	66	250 ml	41	27
Guardian™, breakfast cereal	37	30 g	12	5
Hamburger bun	61	30 g	15	9
Haricot/navy beans, cooked/canned	38*	150 g	31	12
Healthwise™ breakfast cereal for bowel health	66	30 g	18	12
Healthwise™ breakfast cereal for heart health	48	30 g	19	9
Helga's™ Classic Seed Loaf	68	30 g	14	9
Helga's™ traditional wholemeal bread	70	30 g	13	9
Honey, Yellow Box honey	35	25 g	18	6
Honey, Stringybark	44	25 g	21	9
Honey, Ironbark	48	25 g	15	7
Honey, Capilano	64*	25 g	17	11
Honey & Oat bread, Vogel's	55	30 g	14	7
Honey Rice Bubbles™, breakfast cereal	77	30 g	27	20
Honey Smacks™, breakfast cereal	71	30 g	23	11
Ice-cream, Norco, Prestige Light rich Vanilla	47	50 g	10	5
Ice-cream, Norco, Prestige Light Toffee	37	50 g	14	5
Ice-cream, Norco, Prestige Macadamia	39	50 g	12	5
Ice-cream, regular, average	61*	50 g	13	8
Ice-cream, Peter's light and creamy	44	100 ml	14	6
Ice-cream, premium, French vanilla, 16% fat	38	50 g	9	3
Ice-cream, premium, 'ultra chocolate', 15% fat	37	50 g	9	4
Instant mashed potato, prepared	69*	150 g	20	17

* Average

FOOD	GI	NOMINAL SERVE SIZE	AVAILABLE CARB PER SERVE	GL PER SERVE
Instant rice, white, cooked 6 min	87	150 g	42	29
Ironman PR bar®, chocolate	39	65 g	26	10
Isostar® sports drink	70	250 ml	18	13
Jam, apricot fruit spread, reduced sugar	55	30 g	13	7
Jam, strawberry, regular	51	30 g	20	10
Jasmine rice, white, long-grain, cooked in rice cooker	109	150 g	42	46
Jatz™, plain salted cracker biscuits	55	25 g	17	10
Jelly Beans	78*	30 g	28	22
Jevity™, fibre-enriched drink	48	237 ml	36	17
Just Right™, breakfast cereal	60	30 g	22	13
Just Right Just Grains™, breakfast cereal	62	30 g	23	14
Kaiser rolls	73	30 g	16	12
Kavli™ Norwegian Crispbread	71	25 g	16	12
Kidney beans, canned	52	150 g	17	9
Kidz™, Heinz, Fruit Fingers, banana	61	30 g	20	12
Kidney beans, boiled	28*	150 g	25	7
Kiwi fruit, raw	58	120 g	12	7
Komplete™, breakfast cereal	48	30 g	21	10
K-Time Just Right™ breakfast cereal bar	72	30 g	24	17
K-Time Strawberry Crunch™ breakfast cereal bar	77	30 g	25	19
Lactose, pure	46*	10 g	10	5
Lamb	[0]	120 g	0	0
Lamingtons, sponge dipped in chocolate and coconut	87	50 g	29	25
L.E.A.N Fibergy™ bar, Harvest Oat	45	50 g	29	13
L.E.A.N Life long Nutribar™, Peanut Crunch	30	40 g	19	6

* Average

FOOD	GI	NOMINAL SERVE SIZE	AVAILABLE CARB PER SERVE	GL PER SERVE
L.E.A.N Life long Nutribar™, Chocolate Crunch	32	40 g	19	6
L.E.A.N Nutrimeal™, drink powder, Dutch Chocolate	26	250 g	13	3
Lebanese bread, white, I round	75	83 g	45	34
Legumes				
Baked Beans, canned	48*	150 g	17	8
Blackeyed beans, boiled	42*	150 g	21	12
Butter Beans	31	150 g	20	6
Chickpeas, dried, boiled	28*	150 g	24	7
Haricot/navy beans, dried, cooked	38	150 g	31	12
Kidney beans	28	150 g	25	7
Lentils, boiled	29*	150 g	18	5
Lentils, green, dried, boiled	30*	150 g	17	5
Lentils, red, dried, boiled	26*	150 g	18	5
Lima beans	32	150 g	30	10
Marrowfat peas, dried, boiled	39*	150 g	19	7
Mung bean, dried, boiled	31	150 g	17	5
Peas, dried, boiled	22	150 g	9	2
Soy beans, dried, boiled	18*	150 g	6	1
Split peas, yellow, boiled	32	150 g	19	6
Lentils, canned, green	52	50 g	17	9
Lentils, green, dried, boiled	30*	150 g	17	5
Lentils, boiled	29*	150 g	18	5
Lentils, red, boiled	26	150 g	18	5
Life Savers®, peppermint	70	30 g	30	21
Light rye bread	68	30 g	14	10
Lima beans, baby, frozen, reheated in microwave oven	32	150 g	30	10
Linguine pasta, thick, cooked	46*	180 g	48	22
Linguine pasta, thin, cooked	52*	180 g	45	23

* Average

FOOD	GI	NOMINAL SERVE SIZE	AVAILABLE CARB PER SERVE	GL PER SERVE
Lucozade®, original, sparkling glucose drink	95	250 ml	42	40
Lungkow beanthread noodles	26	180 g	45	12
Lychees, canned in syrup, drained	79	120 g	20	16
M & M's®, peanut	33	30 g	17	6
Macaroni, plain, boiled	47*	180 g	48	23
Macaroni and Cheese, made from mix	64	180 g	51	32
Maltose, 50 g	105	10 g	10	11
Mango raw	51*	120 g	17	8
Maple syrup, Pure Canadian	54	24 g	18	10
Marmalade, orange	48	30 g	20	9
Mars Bar®	62	60 g	40	25
Meat				
Beef	[0]	120 g	0	0
Lamb	[0]	120 g	0	0
Pork	[0]	120 g	0	0
Salami	[0]	120 g	0	0
Tuna	[0]	120 g	0	0
Veal	[0]	120 g	0	0
Melba toast	70	30 g	23	16
Milk, full-fat cow's milk, fresh	31	250 ml	12	4
Milk, skim	32	250 ml	13	4
Milk, low fat, chocolate, with sugar, Lite White™	34	250 ml	26	9
Milk, condensed, sweetened	61	50 ml	28	17
Milk Arrowroot™ biscuits	69	25 g	18	12
Milky Bar®, plain, white chocolate	44	50 g	29	13
Millet, boiled	71	150 g	36	25
Milo™, chocolate powder, dissolved in water	54	250 ml	16	9

* Average

FOOD	GI	NOMINAL SERVE SIZE	AVAILABLE CARB PER SERVE	GL PER SERVE
Milo™, ready to drink bottle	30	600 ml	66	20
Mini Wheats™, whole wheat breakfast cereal	58	30 g	21	12
Mini Wheats™, blackcurrant whole wheat breakfast cereal	72	30 g	21	15
Mixed grain loaf, Bürgen®	49*	30 g	11	6
Morning Coffee™, 3 biscuits	79	25 g	19	15
Mousse, butterscotch, reduced fat	36	50 g	10	4
Mousse, chocolate, reduced fat	31	50 g	11	3
Mousse, hazelnut, reduced fat	36	50 g	10	4
Mousse, mango, reduced fat	33	50 g	11	4
Mousse, mixed berry, reduced fat	36	50 g	10	4
Mousse, strawberry, reduced fat	32	50 g	10	3
Muesli bar containing dried fruit	61	30 g	21	13
Muesli, gluten-free with 1.5% fat milk	39	30 g	19	7
Muesli, toasted (Purina)	43	30 g	17	7
Muesli, Swiss Formula, natural	56	30 g	16	9
Multi-Grain 9-Grain	43	30 g	14	6
Mung bean noodles (Lungkow beanthread), dried, boiled	39	180 g	45	18
Nesquik™ powder, chocolate dissolved in 1.5% fat milk	41	250 ml	11	5
Nesquik™ powder, strawberry dissolved in 1.5% fat milk	35	250 ml	12	4
New potato, unpeeled and boiled 20 min	78	150 g	21	16
New potato, canned, heated in microwave 3 min	65	150 g	18	12
No Bake Egg Custard, prepared from powder with whole milk	35	100 ml	17	6
Noodles, instant 'two-minute' Maggi®	47*	180 g	40	19

* Average

FOOD	GI	NOMINAL SERVE SIZE	AVAILABLE CARB PER SERVE	GL PER SERVE
Noodles, mung bean (Lungkow beanthread), dried, boiled	39	180 g	45	18
Noodles, rice, freshly made, boiled	40	180 g	39	15
Norco Ice-cream, Prestige Light rich Vanilla	47	50 g	10	5
Norco Ice-cream, Prestige Light Toffee	37	50 g	14	5
Norco Ice-cream, Prestige Macadamia	39	50 g	12	5
Nutella®, chocolate hazelnut spread	33	20 g	12	4
Nutrigrain™, breakfast cereal	66	30 g	15	10
Oat 'n' Honey Bake™, breakfast cereal	77	30 g	17	13
Oat Bran & Honey Loaf bread, Bürgen®	49	40 g	13	7
Oat bran, raw	55*	10 g	5	3
Orange, 1 medium	42*	120 g	11	5
Orange cordial, reconstituted	66	250 ml	20	13
Orange juice, unsweetened, reconstituted	53	250 ml	18	9
Pancakes, prepared from shake mix	67	70 g	23	15
Pancakes, buckwheat, gluten-free, made from packet mix	102	77 g	22	22
Parsnips	97	80 g	12	12
Party pies, beef, cooked	45	100 g	27	12
Pasta and noodles				
Fettucine, egg, boiled	40*	180 g	46	18
Gnocchi	68	180 g	48	33
Instant noodles	47*	180 g	40	19
Linguine	49*	180 g	47	23
Mung bean noodles	39	180 g	45	18
Macaroni	47	180 g	48	23
Macaroni and Cheese, boxed	64	180 g	51	32

* Average

FOOD	GI	NOMINAL SERVE SIZE	AVAILABLE CARB PER SERVE	GL PER SERVE
Ravioli, meat-filled	39	180 g	38	15
Rice noodles, freshly made	40	180 g	39	15
Rice noodles, dried, boiled	61	180 g	39	23
Rice pasta, brown boiled	92	180 g	38	35
Spaghetti, gluten-free, canned in tomato sauce	68	220 g	27	19
Spaghetti, white, boiled 10-15 min	44*	180 g	48	21
Spaghetti, white, boiled 20 min	61*	180 g	44	27
Spaghetti, white, boiled	42*	180 g	47	20
Spaghetti, wholemeal, boiled	37*	180 g	42	16
Spirali, durum wheat, white, boiled	43	180 g	44	19
Udon noodles, plain	62	180 g	48	30
Pastry, plain	59	57 g	26	15
Paw paw, raw	59*	120 g	8	5
Peach, fresh, 1 large	42*	120 g	11	5
Peach, canned in heavy syrup	58	120 g	15	9
Peach, canned in light syrup	52	120 g	18	9
Peach, canned in reduced-sugar syrup, SPC Lite	62	120 g	17	11
Peanuts, roasted, salted	14*	50 g	6	1
Pear, raw	38*	120 g	11	4
Pear halves, canned in natural juice	43	120 g	13	5
Pear halves, canned in reduced-sugar syrup, (SPC Lite)	25	120 g	14	4
Peas, dried, boiled	22	150 g	9	2
Peas, green, frozen, boiled	48*	80 g	7	3
Pecans (raw)	10	50 g	3	1
Pelde brown rice, boiled	76	150 g	38	29
Performax™ bread	38	30 g	13	5

* Average

FOOD	GI	NOMINAL SERVE SIZE	AVAILABLE CARB PER SERVE	GL PER SERVE
Pikelets, Golden brand	85	40 g	21	18
Pineapple, raw	59*	120 g	10	6
Pineapple juice, unsweetened	46	250 ml	34	15
Pinto beans, canned in brine	45	150 g	22	10
Pinto beans, dried, boiled	39	150 g	26	10
Pita bread, white	57	30 g	17	10
Pizza, cheese	60	100 g	27	16
Pizza, Super Supreme, pan (11.4% fat)	36	100 g	24	9
Pizza, Super Supreme, thin and crispy (13.2 % fat)	30	100 g	22	7
Ploughman's™ Wholegrain bread, original recipe	47	30 g	14	7
Ploughman's™ Wholemeal bread, smooth milled	64	30 g	13	9
Plums, raw	39*	120 g	12	5
Pontiac potato, peeled, boiled 35 min	88	150 g	18	16
Pontiac potato, peeled and microwave on high for 6–7.5 min	79	150 g	18	14
Pontiac potato, peeled, cubed, boiled 15 min, mashed	91	150 g	20	18
Pop Tarts™, Double Chocolate	70	50 g	36	25
Popcorn, plain, cooked in microwave oven	72*	20 g	11	8
Pork	[0]	120 g	0	0
Porridge made from whole oats	55	250 g	21	12
Potato				
Baked potato, Ontario, with skin	60	150 g	30	18
Baked without fat Russet Burbank potato	85*	150 g	30	26
Canned potato, new	65	150 g	18	12
Desiree, peeled, boiled 35 min	101	150 g	17	17
French fries	75	150 g	29	22

* Average

FOOD	GI	NOMINAL SERVE SIZE	AVAILABLE CARB PER SERVE	GL PER SERVE
Instant mashed potato	85	150 g	20	17
New potato	62	150 g	21	13
Ontario, peeled, boiled 35 min	58	150 g	27	16
Pontiac, peeled, boiled 35 min	88	150 g	18	16
Mashed potato				
Pontiac, mashed	91	150 g	20	18
Pontiac, peeled and microwaved on high for 6–7.5 min	79	150 g	18	14
Potato, peeled, steamed	65	150 g	27	18
Sebago, peeled, boiled 35 min	87	150 g	17	14
Sweet potato	44	150 g	25	11
Potato crisps, plain, salted	54*	50 g	21	11
Pound cake	54	53 g	28	15
Power Bar®, chocolate	56*	65 g	42	24
Pretzels, oven-baked, traditional wheat flavour	83	30 g	20	16
Prunes, pitted, 6	29	60 g	33	10
Pudding, instant, chocolate, made from powder and whole milk	47	100 g	16	7
Pudding, instant, vanilla, made from powder and whole milk	40	100 g	16	6
Pudding, Sustagen™, instant vanilla, made from powdered mix	27	250 g	47	13
Puffed crispbread	81	25 g	19	15
Puffed rice cakes, white	82	25 g	21	17
Puffed Wheat, breakfast cereal	80	30 g	21	17
Pumpernickel rye kernel bread	50*	30 g	12	6
Pumpkin	75	80 g	4	3
Quik™, chocolate (Nestlé, Australia), dissolved in 1.5% fat milk	41	250 ml	11	5

* Average

FOOD	GI	NOMINAL SERVE SIZE	AVAILABLE CARB PER SERVE	GL PER SERVE
Quik™, strawberry (Nestlé, Australia), dissolved in 1.5% fat milk	35	250 ml	12	4
Raisins	64	60 g	44	28
Ravioli, durum wheat flour, meat filled, boiled	39	180 g	38	15
Real Fruit Bars, strawberry processed fruit bars	90	30 g	26	23
Rice				
Arborio, risotto rice, boiled	69	150 g	43	29
Basmati, boiled	58	150 g	38	22
Calrose brown	87	150 g	40	35
Calrose, white, medium grain, boiled	83	150 g	42	35
Doongara, brown	66	150 g	37	24
Doongara, white	56	150 g	39	22
Instant Doongara, white	94	150 g	42	35
Instant rice, white	87	150 g	42	36
Jasmine rice, white, long-grain	109	150 g	42	46
Long grain, boiled	56	150 g	41	23
Parboiled, Doongara	50	150 g	39	19
Parboiled, Sungold	87	150 g	39	34
Pelde brown	76	150 g	38	29
Pelde, white	93	150 g	43	40
Rice, brown	55	150 g	33	18
Sunbrown Quick™	80	150 g	38	31
Sungold, Pelde, parboiled	87	150 g	43	37
Rice and maize pasta, Ris'O'Mais, gluten-free	76	180 g	49	37
Rice Bran, extruded	19	30 g	14	3
Rice Bubbles™, breakfast cereal	87	30 g	26	22

* Average

FOOD	GI	NOMINAL SERVE SIZE	AVAILABLE CARB PER SERVE	GL PER SERVE
Rice Bubble Treat™ bar	63	30 g	24	15
Rice cakes, white	82	25 g	21	17
Rice Krispies™, breakfast cereal	82	30 g	26	22
Rice noodles, freshly made, boiled	40	180 g	39	15
Rice pasta, brown, boiled 16 min	92	180 g	38	35
Rice vermicelli, dried, boiled	58	180 g	39	22
Rich Tea, 2 biscuits	55	25 g	19	10
Risotto rice, arborio, boiled	69	150 g	43	29
Rockmelon/cantaloupe, raw	65	120 g	6	4
Roggenbrot, Vogel's	59	30 g	14	8
Roll (bread), Kaiser	73	30 g	16	12
Roll-Ups®, processed fruit snack	99	30 g	25	24
Romano beans	46	150 g	18	8
Rye bread, wholemeal	58*	30 g	14	8
Ryvita™ crackers	69	25 g	16	11
Salami	[0]	120 g	0	0
Salmon	0	150 g	0	0
Sao™, plain square crackers	70	25 g	17	12
Sausages, fried	28	100 g	3	1
Scones, plain, made from packet mix	92	25 g	9	8
Sebago potato, peeled, boiled 35 min	87	150 g	17	14
Semolina cooked	55*	150 g	11	6
Shellfish (prawns, crab, lobster etc)	[0]	120 g	0	0
Shortbread biscuits	64	25 g	16	10
Shredded Wheat, breakfast cereal	75*	30 g	20	15
Shredded Wheatmeal™ biscuits	62	25 g	18	11
Skittles®	70	50 g	45	32
Snack foods				
Apricot filled fruit bar	50	50 g	34	17
Burger Rings™	90	50 g	31	28
Chocolate, milk, plain	43	50 g	28	12

* Average

FOOD	GI	NOMINAL SERVE SIZE	AVAILABLE CARB PER SERVE	GL PER SERVE
Chocolate, white, Milky Bar®	44	50 g	29	13
Corn chips, plain, salted	42	50 g	25	11
Heinz Kidz™ Fruit Fingers, banana	61	30 g	20	12
Fruity Bitz™	39	15 g	12	4
Jelly beans	78	30 g	28	22
Life Savers®, peppermint	70	30 g	30	21
M & M's®, peanut	33	30 g	17	6
Mars Bar®	62	60 g	40	25
Muesli bar with dried fruit	61	30 g	21	13
Nutella®	33	20 g	12	4
Popcorn, cooked in microwave	72	20 g	11	8
Pop Tarts™, chocolate	70	50 g	35	24
Potato crisps, plain, salted	57	50 g	18	10
Pretzels	83	30 g	20	16
Real Fruit Bars, strawberry	90	30 g	26	23
Roll-Ups®	99	30 g	25	24
Skittles®	70	50 g	45	32
Snickers Bar®	41	60 g	36	15
Twisties™, cheese flavoured	74	50 g	29	22
Twix®	44	60 g	39	17
So Natural™ soy milk, full-fat (3%), 120 mg calcium, Calciforte	36	250 ml	18	6
So Natural™ soy milk, reduced-fat (1.5%), 120 mg calcium, Light	44	250 ml	17	8
So Natural™ soy milk, full-fat (3%), 0 mg calcium, Original	44	250 ml	17	8
So Natural™ soy smoothie drink, banana, 1% fat	30	250 ml	22	7
So Natural™ soy smoothie drink, chocolate hazelnut, 1% fat	34	250 ml	25	8

* Average

FOOD	GI	NOMINAL SERVE SIZE	AVAILABLE CARB PER SERVE	GL PER SERVE
So Natural™ soy yoghurt, peach and mango, 2% fat, sugar	50	200 ml	26	13
Soft drinks				
Coca Cola®, soft drink	53	250 ml	26	14
Cordial, orange	66	250 ml	20	13
Fanta®, orange soft drink	68	250 ml	34	23
Lucozade®, original	95	250 ml	42	40
Solo™, lemon squash, soft drink	58	250 ml	29	17
Soups				
Black Bean	64	250 ml	27	17
Green Pea, canned	66	250 ml	41	27
Lentil, canned	44	250 ml	21	9
Minestrone, Country Ladle™	39	250 ml	18	7
Split Pea	60	250 ml	27	16
Tomato soup	38	250 ml	17	6
Sourdough rye	48	30 g	12	6
Sourdough wheat	54	30 g	14	8
Soy milk, So Natural™ full-fat (3%), 120 mg calcium, Calciforte	36	250 ml	18	6
Soy milk, So Natural™ reduced-fat (1.5%), 120 mg calcium, Light	44	250 ml	17	8
Soy milk, So Natural™ full-fat (3%), 0 mg calcium, Original	44	250 ml	17	8
Soy smoothie drink, So Natural™ banana, 1% fat	30	250 ml	22	7
Soy smoothie drink, So Natural™ chocolate hazelnut, 1% fat	34	250 ml	25	8
Soy yoghurt, So Natural™ peach and mango, 2% fat, sugar	50	200 g	26	13
Soy beans, dried, boiled	18*	150 g	6	1
Soy beans, canned	14	150 g	6	1

* Average

FOOD	GI	NOMINAL SERVE SIZE	AVAILABLE CARB PER SERVE	GL PER SERVE
Soy-Lin, Bürgen® kibbled soy (8%) and linseed (8%) bread	36	30 g	9	3
Spaghetti, gluten-free, rice and split pea, canned in tomato sauce	68	220 g	27	19
Spaghetti, white, boiled 5 minutes	38*	180 g	48	18
Spaghetti, wholemeal, boiled 5 minutes	37	180 g	42	16
Special K™, breakfast cereal	54	30 g	21	11
Spirali pasta, durum wheat, white, boiled to al denté texture	43	180 g	44	19
Split pea and soy pasta shells, gluten-free	29	180 g	31	9
Split Pea soup	60	250 ml	27	16
Split peas, yellow, boiled 20 min	32	150 g	19	6
Sponge cake, plain	46	63 g	36	17
Sports drinks				
Gatorade®	78	250 ml	15	12
Isostar®	70	250 ml	18	13
Sports Plus®	74	250 ml	17	13
Sustagen Sport®	43	250 ml	49	21
Sports Plus®, sport drink	74	250 ml	17	13
Stoned Wheat Thins crackers	67	25 g	17	12
Strawberries, fresh	40	120 g	3	1
Strawberry jam, regular	51	30 g	20	10
Stuffing, bread	74	30 g	21	16
Sucrose	68*	10 g	10	7
Sugars and honey				
Fructose	19*	10 g	10	2
Glucose	100	10 g	10	10
Iron Bark honey	48	25 g	15	7
Lactose	46*	10 g	10	5
Maltose	105	10 g	10	11

* Average

FOOD	GI	NOMINAL SERVE SIZE	AVAILABLE CARB PER SERVE	GL PER SERVE
Pure Capilano™ honey	58	25 g	21	12
Red Gum honey	46	25 g	18	8
Salvation Jane honey	64	25 g	15	10
Stringy Bark honey	44	25 g	21	9
Sucrose	68*	10 g	10	7
Yapunya honey	52	25 g	17	9
Yellow box honey	35	25 g	18	6
Sultana Bran™, breakfast cereal	73	30 g	19	14
Sultanas	56	60 g	45	25
Sunbrown Quick™ rice, boiled	80	150 g	38	31
Sunflower and barley bread, (Riga)	57	30 g	11	6
Super Supreme pizza, pan (11.4% fat)	36	100 g	24	9
Super Supreme pizza, thin and crispy (13.2% fat)	30	100 g	22	7
Sushi, salmon	48	100 g	36	17
Sustagen™ Hospital with extra fibre, drink made from powdered mix	33	250 ml	44	15
Sustagen™ drink, Dutch Chocolate	31	250 ml	41	13
Sustagen™ pudding, instant vanilla, made from powdered mix	27	250 ml	47	13
Sustagen Sport®, milk-based drink	43	250 ml	49	21
Sustain™, breakfast cereal	68	30 g	22	15
Sustain™ cereal bar	57	30 g	25	14
Swede, cooked	72	150 g	10	7
Sweet corn, whole kernel, canned, drained	46	80 g	14	7
Sweet corn on the cob, boiled	48	80 g	16	8
Sweet potato, cooked	44	150 g	25	11
Sweetened condensed whole milk	61	50 g	28	17
Taco shells, cornmeal-based, baked	68	20 g	12	8
Tapioca, boiled with milk	81	250 ml	18	14

* Average

FOOD	GI	NOMINAL SERVE SIZE	AVAILABLE CARB PER SERVE	GL PER SERVE
Tomato soup	38	250 ml	17	6
Tortellini, cheese, cooked	50	180 g	21	10
TRIM™ custard, reduced-fat	37	100 g	15	6
Tuna	[0]	120 g	0	0
Twisties™, cheese-flavoured, extruded snack, rice and corn	74	50 g	29	22
Twix® Bar, caramel	44	60 g	39	17
Ultra chocolate ice-cream, premium 15% fat (Sara Lee)	37	50 g	9	4
Vaalia™, reduced-fat apricot and mango yoghurt	26	200 g	30	8
Vaalia™, reduced-fat French vanilla yoghurt	26	200 g	10	3
Yoghurt, no-fat, French vanilla, Vaalia, with sugar	40	150 ml	27	10
Yoghurt, no-fat, Mango, Vaalia, with sugar	39	150 ml	25	10
Yoghurt, no-fat, Wildberry, Vaalia, with sugar	38	150 ml	22	8
Yoghurt, no-fat, Strawberry, Vaalia, with sugar	38	150 ml	22	8
Vaalia™, reduced-fat tropical passionfruit yoghurt drink	38	200 ml	29	11
Vanilla cake made from packet mix with vanilla frosting	42	111 g	58	24
Vanilla pudding, instant, made from packet mix and whole milk	40	100 g	16	6
Vanilla wafers, 6 biscuits	77	25 g	18	14
Veal	[0]	120 g	0	0
Vegetables				
Artichokes	[0]	80 g	0	0
Avocado	[0]	80 g	0	0

* Average

FOOD	GI	NOMINAL SERVE SIZE	AVAILABLE CARB PER SERVE	GL PER SERVE
Beetroot	64	80 g	7	5
Bokchoy	[0]	80 g	0	0
Broad beans	79	80 g	11	9
Broccoli	[0]	80 g	0	0
Cabbage	[0]	80 g	0	0
Carrots, peeled, boiled	41*	80 g	5	2
Capsicum	[0]	80 g	0	0
Cauliflower	[0]	80 g	0	0
Celery	[0]	80 g	0	0
Corn on the cob, sweet, boiled	48	80 g	16	8
Cucumber	[0]	80 g	0	0
French beans (runner beans)	[0]	80 g	0	0
Green peas	48	80 g	7	3
Leafy vegetables (spinach, rocket etc)	[0]	80 g	0	0
Lettuce	[0]	80 g	0	0
Parsnips, boiled	97	80 g	12	12
Vermicelli, white, boiled	35	180 g	44	16
Vita-Brits™, breakfast cereal	68	30 g	20	13
Vitari, wild berry, non-dairy, frozen fruit dessert	59	100 g	21	12
Vogel's Honey & Oats bread	55	30 g	14	7
Waffles	76	35 g	13	10
Water crackers	78	25 g	18	14
Watermelon, raw	72	120 g	6	4
Weis Mango Frutia™, low fat frozen fruit dessert	42	100 g	23	10
Weet-Bix™, breakfast cereal	69	30 g	17	12
Wheat-bites™, breakfast cereal	72	30 g	25	18
White bread, wheat flour	70	30 g	14	10
Wholemeal bread, wheat flour	71*	30 g	12	9

* Average

FOOD	GI	NOMINAL SERVE SIZE	AVAILABLE CARB PER SERVE	GL PER SERVE
Wholemeal, sandwich bread (Tip Top)	70	59 g	24	17
Wild About Fruit Apple Juice, pure, clear, unsweetened	44	250 ml	30	13
Wild About Fruit Apple Juice, pure, cloudy, unsweetened	37	250 ml	28	10
Wild About Fruit Apple and mandarin juice	53	250 ml	29	15
Wild About Fruit Apple and mango juice	44	250 ml	27	12
Wonderwhite™ bread	80	30 g	14	11
Yam, peeled, boiled	37*	150 g	36	13
Yoghurt, diet, low fat, no added sugar, vanilla	23	200 ml	13	3
Yoghurt, diet, low fat, no added sugar, (fruit)	24*	200 ml	13	3
Yoghurt drink, Vaalia™, reduced-fat tropical passionfruit	38	200 ml	29	11
Yoghurt, low fat, fruit with artificial sweetener	14	200 ml	13	2
Yoghurt, low fat, fruit with sugar	33	200 ml	31	10
Yoghurt, low fat (0.9%), wild strawberry	31	200 ml	30	9
Yoghurt, no-fat, French vanilla, Vaalia, with sugar	40	150 ml	27	10
Yoghurt, no-fat, Mango, Vaalia, with sugar	39	150 ml	25	10
Yoghurt, no-fat, Wildberry, Vaalia, with sugar	38	150 ml	22	8
Yoghurt, no-fat, Strawberry, Vaalia, with sugar	38	150 ml	22	8

* Average

FOOD CATEGORY
GI VALUES

Many of our readers have asked for GI values to be listed in food categories rather than in A to Z format, for easier access. The categories include: bakery products; beverages; breads; breakfast cereals and bars; cereal grains; cookies; crackers; dairy products; fruit and fruit products; infant formulas; legumes and nuts; meal replacement products; mixed meals and convenience foods; nutritional support products; pasta and noodles; protein foods; snack foods and confectionary; sports bars; soups; sugars; and vegetables.

Within food categories, we have grouped the foods in alphabetical order to help you choose the low GI versions within each category ('this for that') and also to mix and match. If your favourite food has a high GI, check out its glycemic load. If that's relatively low compared with other foods in that group, then you don't have to worry unduly about its high GI. If it's both high GI and high GL try to cut down the serving size or team it with a very low GI food (e.g. rice (high GI) and lentils (low GI)).

In this food category listing, we have included all the data available, not just average figures and not just Australian data. Here you will find GI values from all over the world, including the United States, Canada, New Zealand, Italy, Sweden, Japan and China among others. Australians are lucky to have more of their foods tested than any other country.

As with the A to Z listing we have also included foods that have very little carbohydrate and were omitted from previous editions. However, since so many people ask us for the GI of these foods, we decided to include them and show their GI as [0].

Note: NS means that a brand was not specified.

FOOD	GI	NOMINAL SERVE SIZE	AVAILABLE CARB PER SERVE	GL PER SERVE
BAKERY PRODUCTS				
Cakes				
Angel food cake (Loblaw's, Toronto, Canada)	67	50 g	29	19
Banana cake, home made with sugar	47	80 g	38	18
Banana cake, home made without sugar	55	80 g	29	16
Chocolate cake, made from packet mix with chocolate frosting (Betty Crocker)	38	111 g	52	20
Crumpet	69	50 g	19	13
Cupcake, strawberry-iced	73	38 g	26	19
Doughnut, cake type	76	47 g	23	17
Flan cake	65	70 g	48	31
Lamingtons (sponge dipped in chocolate and coconut)	87	50 g	29	25
Pancakes, prepared from shake mix	67	70 g	23	15
Pancakes, buckwheat, gluten-free, made from packet mix (Orgran)	102	77 g	22	22
Pikelets, Golden brand (Tip Top)	85	40 g	21	18
Pound cake (Sara Lee)	54	53 g	28	15
Scones, plain, made from packet mix	92	25 g	9	8
Sponge cake, plain	46	63 g	36	17
Vanilla cake, made from packet mix with vanilla frosting (Betty Crocker)	42	111 g	58	24
Waffles, Aunt Jemima	76	35 g	13	10
Muffins				
Apple, made with sugar	44	60 g	29	13
Apple, made without sugar	48	60 g	19	9

* Average

FOOD	GI	NOMINAL SERVE SIZE	AVAILABLE CARB PER SERVE	GL PER SERVE
Apple, oat, sultana, made from packet mix	54	50 g	26	14
Apricot, coconut and honey, made from packet mix	60	50 g	26	16
Banana, oat and honey, made from packet mix	65	50 g	26	17
Blueberry muffin	59	57 g	29	17
Bran	60	57 g	24	15
Carrot muffin	62	57 g	32	20
Chocolate butterscotch, made from packet mix	53	50 g	28	15
Oatmeal, muffin, made from mix (Quaker Oats)	69	50 g	35	24
Pastry				
Croissant	67	57 g	26	17
Pastry	59	57 g	26	15

BEVERAGES

Alcoholic beverages				
Beer	[0]	250 ml	10	0
Brandy	[0]	30 ml	0	0
Gin	[0]	30 ml	0	0
Red wine	[0]	100 ml	0	0
Sherry	[0]	60 ml	0	0
Whisky	[0]	30 ml	0	0
White wine	[0]	100 ml	0	0
Juices				
Apple juice, pure, unsweetened, (Bern) (Australia)	39			
Apple juice, unsweetened (USA)	40			
Apple juice, unsweetened (Canada)	41			

* Average

FOOD	GI	NOMINAL SERVE SIZE	AVAILABLE CARB PER SERVE	GL PER SERVE
Average of three studies	40	250 ml	29	12
Apple juice, pure, clear, unsweetened (Wild About Fruit, Australia)	44	250 ml	30	13
Apple juice, pure, cloudy, unsweetened (Wild About Fruit, Australia)	37	250 ml	28	10
Carrot juice, freshly made (Sydney, Australia)	43	250 ml	23	10
Cranberry juice cocktail (Ocean Spray®, Australia)	52	250 ml	31	16
Cranberry juice cocktail (Ocean Spray®, USA)	68	250 ml	36	24
Cranberry juice drink (Ocean Spray®, UK)	56	250 ml	29	16
Grapefruit juice, unsweetened (Sunpac, Canada)	48	250 ml	22	11
Orange juice (Canada)	46	250 ml	26	12
Orange juice, unsweetened, (Quelch®, Australia)	53	250 ml	18	9
Pineapple juice, unsweetened (Dole, Canada)	46	250 ml	34	16
Tomato juice, canned, no added sugar (Berri, Australia)	38	250 ml	9	4
Powder drinks				
Build-Up™ with fiber, (Nestlé)	41	250 ml	33	14
Complete Hot Chocolate mix with hot water (Nestlé)	51	250 ml	23	11
Hi-Pro energy drink mix, vanilla, (Harrod)	36	250 ml	19	7
Malted milk in full-fat cow's milk (Nestlé, Australia)	45	250 ml	26	12

* Average

FOOD	GI	NOMINAL SERVE SIZE	AVAILABLE CARB PER SERVE	GL PER SERVE
Milo™ (chocolate nutrient-fortified drink powder)				
Milo™ (Nestlé, Australia), in water	55	250 ml	16	9
Milo™ (Nestlé, Auckland, New Zealand), in water	52	250 ml	16	9
Milo™ (Nestlé, Australia), in full-fat cow's milk	35	250 ml	25	9
Milo™ (Nestlé, New Zealand), in full-fat cow's milk	36	250 ml	26	9
Milo™, (Nestlé, Australia), bottle	30	600 ml	64	19
Milo™, (Nestlé, Australia), tetrapak	35	250 ml	31	11
Nutrimeal™, meal replacement drink, Dutch Chocolate (Usana)	26	250 ml	17	4
Quik™, chocolate (Nestlé, Australia), in water	53	250 ml	7	4
Quik™, chocolate (Nestlé, Australia), in 1.5% fat milk	41	250 ml	11	5
Quik™, strawberry (Nestlé, Australia), in water	64	250 ml	8	5
Quik™, strawberry (Nestlé, Australia), in 1.5% fat milk	35	250 ml	12	4
Smoothies and shakes				
Smoothie, raspberry (Con Agra)	33	250 ml	41	14
Smoothie drink, soy, banana (So Natural)	30	250 ml	22	7
Smoothie drink, soy, chocolate hazelnut (So Natural)	34	250 ml	25	8
Up & Go, cocoa malt flavor (Sanitarium)	43	250 ml	26	11
Up & Go, original malt flavor (Sanitarium)	46	250 ml	24	11

* Average

FOOD	GI	NOMINAL SERVE SIZE	AVAILABLE CARB PER SERVE	GL PER SERVE
Xpress™ chocolate (So Natural, Australia)	39	250 ml	34	13
Yakult® (Yakult, Australia)	46	65 ml	12	6
Soft drinks				
Coca Cola®, soft drink (Australia)	53	250 ml	26	14
Coca Cola®, soft drink/soda (USA)	63	250 ml	26	16
Cordial, orange, reconstituted (Berri)	66	250 ml	20	13
Fanta®, orange soft drink (Australia)	68	250 ml	34	23
Lucozade®, original (sparkling glucose drink)	95	250 ml	42	40
Solo™, lemon squash, soft drink (Australia)	58	250 ml	29	17
Sports drinks				
Gatorade® (Australia)	78	250 ml	15	12
Isostar® (Switzerland)	70	250 ml	18	13
Sports Plus® (Australia)	74	250 ml	17	13
Sustagen Sport® (Australia)	43	250 ml	49	21

BREADS

FOOD	GI	NOMINAL SERVE SIZE	AVAILABLE CARB PER SERVE	GL PER SERVE
Bagel, white, frozen (Canada)	72	70 g	35	25
Baguette, white, plain (France)	95	30 g	15	14
French baguette with chocolate spread (France)	72	70 g	37	27
French baguette with butter and strawberry jam (France)	62	70 g	41	26
Pain au lait (Pasquier, France)	63	60 g	32	20
Bread stuffing, Paxo (Canada)	74	30 g	21	16
Barley flour breads				
100% barley flour (Canada)	67	30 g	13	9
Sunflower and barley bread (Riga, Sydney, Australia)	57	30 g	11	6

* Average

FOOD	GI	NOMINAL SERVE SIZE	AVAILABLE CARB PER SERVE	GL PER SERVE
Fruit Breads				
Fruit and Spice Loaf, thick sliced (Buttercup, Australia)	54	30 g	15	8
Continental fruit loaf, wheat bread with dried fruit (Australia)	47	30 g	15	7
Happiness™ (cinnamon, raisin, pecan bread) (Natural Ovens, USA)	63	30 g	14	9
Muesli bread, made from packet mix in bread oven (Con Agra, USA)	54	30 g	12	7
Gluten-free Bread				
Gluten-free multigrain bread (Country Life Bakeries, Australia)	79	30 g	13	10
Gluten-free white bread, unsliced (gluten-free wheat starch) (UK)	71	30 g	15	11
Gluten-free white bread, sliced (gluten-free wheat starch) (UK)	80	30 g	15	12
mean of two UK studies	76	30 g	15	11
Gluten-free fibre-enriched, unsliced (gluten-free wheat starch, soya bran) (UK)	69	30 g	13	9
Gluten-free fibre-enriched, sliced (gluten-free wheat starch, soya bran) (UK)	76	30 g	13	10
mean of two studies	73	30 g	13	9
Rice Bread				
Rice bread, low-amylose Calrose rice (Pav's, Australia)	72	30 g	12	8
Rice bread, high-amylose Doongara rice (Pav's, Australia)	61	30 g	12	7
Rolls				
Hamburger bun (Loblaw's, Toronto, Canada)	61	30 g	15	9

* Average

FOOD	GI	NOMINAL SERVE SIZE	AVAILABLE CARB PER SERVE	GL PER SERVE
Kaiser rolls (Loblaw's, Canada)	73	30 g	16	12
Rye Bread (pumpernickel)				
Rye kernel bread (Pumpernickel) (Canada)	41	30 g	12	5
Wholegrain pumpernickel (Holtzheuser Brothers Ltd., Toronto, Canada)	46	30 g	11	5
Rye kernel bread, pumpernickel (80% kernels) (Canada)	55	30 g	12	7
Cocktail, sliced (Kasselar Food Products, Toronto, Canada)	55	30 g	12	7
Cocktail, sliced (Kasselar Food Products, Canada)	62	30 g	12	8
Average of six studies	50	30 g	12	6
Wholemeal rye bread	58	30 g	14	8
Specialty rye breads				
Blackbread, Riga (Berzin's, Sydney, Australia)	76	30 g	13	10
Bürgen™ Dark/Swiss rye (Tip Top Bakeries, Australia)	65	30 g	10	7
Klosterbrot wholemeal rye bread (Dimpflmeier, Canada)	67	30 g	13	9
Light rye (Silverstein's, Canada)	68	30 g	14	10
Linseed rye (Rudolph's, Canada)	55	30 g	13	7
Roggenbrot, Vogel's (Stevns & Co, Sydney, Australia)	59	30 g	14	8
Schinkenbrot, Riga (Berzin's, Sydney, Australia)	86	30 g	14	12
Sourdough rye (Canada)	57			
Sourdough rye (Australia)	48			
Average of two studies	53	30 g	12	6

* Average

FOOD	GI	NOMINAL SERVE SIZE	AVAILABLE CARB PER SERVE	GL PER SERVE
Volkornbrot, wholemeal rye bread (Dimpflmeier, Canada)	56	30 g	13	7
Wheat Breads				
Coarse wheat kernel bread, 80% intact kernels (Sweden)	52	30 g	20	10
Spelt wheat breads				
White spelt wheat bread (Slovenia)	74	30 g	23	17
Wholemeal spelt wheat bread (Slovenia)	63	30 g	19	12
Scalded spelt wheat kernel bread (Slovenia)	67	30 g	22	15
Spelt multigrain bread® (Pav's, Australia)	54	30 g	12	7
White wheat flour bread				
White flour (Canada)	69	30 g	14	10
White flour (USA)	70	30 g	14	10
White flour, Sunblest™ (Tip Top, Australia)	70	30 g	14	10
White flour (Dempster's Corporate Foods Ltd., Canada)	71	30 g	14	10
White flour (South Africa)	71	30 g	13	9
White flour (Canada)	71	30 g	14	10
mean of six studies	70	30 g	14	10
White wheat flour bread, hard, toasted (Italian)	73	30 g	15	11
Wonder™, enriched white bread (USA)	73	30 g	14	10
White Turkish bread (Turkey)	87	30 g	17	15
White bread eaten with vinegar as vinaigrette (Sweden)	45	30 g	15	7
White bread eaten with powdered dried seaweed	48	30 g	15	7

* Average

FOOD	GI	NOMINAL SERVE SIZE	AVAILABLE CARB PER SERVE	GL PER SERVE
White bread containing Eurylon® high-amylose maize starch (France)	42	30 g	19	8
White fibre-enriched bread				
White, high-fibre (Dempster's, Canada)	67			
White, high-fibre (Weston's Bakery, Toronto, Canada)	69			
mean of two studies	68	30 g	13	9
White resistant starch-enriched bread				
Fibre White™ (Nature's Fresh, New Zealand)	77	30 g	15	11
Wonderwhite™ (Buttercup, Australia)	80	30 g	14	11
Wholemeal (whole wheat) wheat flour bread				
Wholemeal flour (Canada)	66*	30 g	12	8
Wholemeal flour (USA)	73	30 g	14	10
Wholemeal flour (South Africa)	75	30 g	13	9
Wholemeal flour (Tip Top Bakeries, Australia)	78	30 g	12	9
Wholemeal flour (Kenya)	87	30 g	13	11
Wholemeal Turkish bread	49	30 g	16	8
Specialty wheat breads				
Bürgen® Mixed Grain (Tip Top, Australia)	49*	30 g	11	6
Bürgen® Oat Bran & Honey (Tip Top, Australia)	49	40 g	13	7
Bürgen® Soy-Lin, kibbled soy (8%) and linseed (8%) loaf (Tip Top)	36	30 g	9	3
English Muffin™ bread (Natural Ovens, USA)	77	30 g	14	11

* Average

FOOD	GI	NOMINAL SERVE SIZE	AVAILABLE CARB PER SERVE	GL PER SERVE
Healthy Choice™ Hearty 7 Grain (Con Agra Inc., USA)	55	30 g	14	8
Healthy Choice™ Hearty 100% Whole Grain (Con Agra Inc., USA)	62	30 g	14	9
Helga's™ Classic Seed Loaf (Quality Bakers, Australia)	68	30 g	14	9
Helga's™ traditional wholemeal bread (Quality Bakers, Australia)	70	30 g	13	9
Holsom's wholemeal and rye	63	74 g	28	18
Holsom's sunflower and poppyseed	61	74 g	30	18
Hunger Filler™, whole grain bread (Natural Ovens, USA)	59	30 g	13	7
Molenberg™ (Goodman Fielder, Auckland, New Zealand)	80	30 g	14	11
9 Grain-Multigrain (Tip Top, Australia)	43	30 g	14	6
Nutty Natural™, whole grain bread (Natural Ovens, USA)	59	30 g	12	7
Performax™ (Country Life Bakeries, Australia)	38	30 g	13	5
Ploughman's™ Wholegrain, original recipe (Quality Bakers, Australia)	47	30 g	14	7
Ploughman's™ Wholemeal, smooth milled (Quality Bakers, Australia)	64	30 g	13	9
Semolina Bread (Kenya)	64			
Sourdough wheat (Australia)	54	30 g	14	8
Soy & Linseed bread (packet mix in bread oven) (Con Agra Inc., USA)	50	30 g	10	5
Stay Trim™, whole grain bread (Natural Ovens, USA)	70	30 g	15	10
Sunflower & Barley bread, Riga brand (Berzin's, Australia)	57	30 g	13	7

* Average

FOOD	GI	NOMINAL SERVE SIZE	AVAILABLE CARB PER SERVE	GL PER SERVE
Vogel's Honey & Oats (Stevns & Co., Australia)	55	30 g	14	7
Vogel's Roggenbrot (Stevns & Co., Australia)	59	30 g	14	8
Whole-wheat snack bread (Ryvita Co Ltd., UK)	74	30 g	22	16
100% Whole Grain™ bread (Natural Ovens, USA)	51	30 g	13	7
Unleavened Breads				
Lebanese bread, white (Seda Bakery, Australia)	75	30 g	16	12
Middle Eastern flatbread	97	30 g	16	15
Pita bread, white (Canada)	57	30 g	17	10
Wheat flour flatbread (India)	66	30 g	16	10
Amaranth : wheat (25:75) composite flour flatbread (India)	66	30 g	15	10
Amaranth : wheat (50:50) composite flour flatbread (India)	76	30 g	15	11

BREAKFAST CEREALS AND RELATED PRODUCTS

FOOD	GI	NOMINAL SERVE SIZE	AVAILABLE CARB PER SERVE	GL PER SERVE
All-Bran™ (Kellogg's, Australia)	30	30 g	15	4
All-Bran™ (Kellogg's, USA)	38	30 g	23	9
All-Bran™ (Kellogg's Inc., Canada)	51	30 g	23	9
Average of three studies	40	30 g	21	8
All-Bran Fruit 'n' Oats™ (Kellogg's, Australia)	39	30 g	17	7
All-Bran Soy 'n' Fibre™ (Kellogg's, Australia)	33	30 g	14	4
Amaranth, popped, with milk (India)	97	30 g	19	18
Bran Buds™ (Kellogg's, Canada)	58	30 g	12	7

* Average

FOOD	GI	NOMINAL SERVE SIZE	AVAILABLE CARB PER SERVE	GL PER SERVE
Bran Buds with psyllium (Kellogg's, Canada)	47	30 g	12	6
Bran Chex™ (Nabisco, Canada)	58	30 g	19	11
Bran Flakes™ (Kellogg's, Australia)	74	30 g	18	13
Cheerios™ (General Mills, Canada)	74	30 g	20	15
Chocapic™ (Nestlé, France)	84	30 g	25	21
Coco Pops™ (Kellogg's, Australia)	77	30 g	26	20
Corn Bran™ (Quaker Oats, Canada)	75	30 g	20	15
Corn Chex™ (Nabisco, Canada)	83	30 g	25	21
Cornflakes™ (Kellogg's, New Zealand)	72	30 g	25	18
Cornflakes™ (Kellogg's, Australia)	77	30 g	25	20
Cornflakes™ (Kellogg's, Canada)	83*	30 g	26	22
Cornflakes™ (Kellogg's, USA)	92	30 g	26	24
Average of four studies	81	30 g	26	21
Cornflakes, high-fibre (Presidents Choice, Canada)	74	30 g	23	17
Cornflakes, Crunchy Nut™ (Kellogg's, Australia)	72	30 g	24	17
Corn Pops™ (Kellogg's, Australia)	80	30 g	26	21
Cream of Wheat™ (Nabisco, Canada)	66	250 g	26	17
Cream of Wheat™, Instant (Nabisco, Canada)	74	250 g	30	22
Crispix™ (Kellogg's, Canada)	87	30 g	25	22
Energy Mix™ (Quaker, France)	80	30 g	24	19
Froot Loops™ (Kellogg's, Australia)	69	30 g	26	18
Frosties™, sugar-coated cornflakes (Kellogg's, Australia)	55	30 g	26	15
Fruitful Lite™ (Hubbards, New Zealand)	61	30 g	20	12

* Average

FOOD	GI	NOMINAL SERVE SIZE	AVAILABLE CARB PER SERVE	GL PER SERVE
Fruity-Bix™, berry (Sanitarium, New Zealand)	113	30 g	22	25
Golden Grahams™ (General Mills, Canada)	71	30 g	25	18
Golden Wheats™ (Kellogg's, Australia)	71	30 g	23	16
Grapenuts™ (Post, Kraft, Canada)	67	30 g	19	13
Grapenuts™ (Kraft, USA)	75	30 g	22	16
Average of two studies	71	30 g	21	15
Grapenuts™ Flakes (Post, Canada)	80	30 g	22	17
Guardian™ (Kellogg's, Australia)	37	30 g	12	5
Healthwise™ for bowel health (Uncle Toby's, Australia)	66	30 g	18	12
Healthwise™ for heart health (Uncle Toby's, Australia)	48	30 g	19	9
Honey Rice Bubbles™ (Kellogg's, Australia)	77	30 g	27	20
Honey Smacks™ (Kellogg's, Australia)	71	30 g	23	16
Hot cereal, apple & cinnamon (Con Agra Inc., USA)	37	30 g	22	8
Hot cereal, unflavoured (Con Agra Inc., USA)	25	30 g	19	5
Just Right™ (Kellogg's, Australia)	60	30 g	22	13
Just Right Just Grains™ (Kellogg's, Australia)	62	30 g	23	14
Komplete™ (Kellogg's, Australia)	48	30 g	21	10
Life™ (Quaker Oats Co., Canada)	66	30 g	25	16
Mini Wheats™, whole wheat (Kellogg's, Australia)	58	30 g	21	12
Mini Wheats™, blackcurrant (Kellogg's, Australia)	72	30 g	21	15

* Average

FOOD	GI	NOMINAL SERVE SIZE	AVAILABLE CARB PER SERVE	GL PER SERVE
Muesli (Canada)	66	30 g	24	16
Alpen Muesli (Wheetabix, France)	55	30 g	19	10
Muesli, gluten-free (Freedom Foods, Australia)	39	30 g	19	7
Muesli, Lite (Sanitarium, New Zealand)	54	30 g	18	10
Muesli, Natural (Sanitarium, New Zealand)	57	30 g	19	11
Muesli, Natural (Sanitarium, Australia)	40	30 g	19	8
Muesli, No Name (Sunfresh, Canada)	60	30 g	18	11
Muesli, Swiss Formula (Uncle Toby's, Australia)	56	30 g	16	9
Muesli, toasted (Purina, Australia)	43	30 g	17	7
Nutrigrain™ (Kellogg's, Australia)	66	30 g	15	10
Oat 'n' Honey Bake™ (Kellogg's, Australia)	77	30 g	17	13
Oat bran, raw (Quaker Oats, Canada)	50	10 g	5	2
Oat bran, raw	59	10 g	5	3
Average of two studies	55	10 g	5	3
Porridge (Uncle Toby's, Australia)	42	250 g	21	9
Porridge (Canada)	49	250 g	23	11
Traditional porridge oats (Lowan, Australia)	51	250 g	21	11
Porridge (Hubbards, New Zealand)	58	250 g	21	12
Porridge (Australia)	58	250 g	21	12
Porridge (Canada)	62	250 g	23	14
Porridge (Canada)	69	250 g	23	16
Porridge (USA)	75	250 g	23	17
Average of eight studies	58	250 g	22	13
Quick Oats (Quaker Oats, Canada)	65	250 g	26	17

* Average

65

FOOD	GI	NOMINAL SERVE SIZE	AVAILABLE CARB PER SERVE	GL PER SERVE
One Minute Oats (Quaker Oats, Canada)	66	250 g	26	17
Average of two studies	66	250 g	26	17
Pop Tarts™, Double Chocolate (Kellogg's, Australia)	70	50 g	36	25
Pro Stars™ (General Mills, Canada)	71	30 g	24	17
Puffed Wheat (Quaker Oats, Canada)	67	30 g	20	13
Puffed Wheat (Sanitarium, Australia)	80	30 g	21	17
Average of two studies	74	30 g	21	16
Raisin Bran™ (Kellogg's, USA)	61	30 g	19	12
Red River Cereal (Maple Leaf Mills, Canada)	49	30 g	22	11
Rice Bran, extruded (Rice Growers, Australia)	19	30 g	14	3
Rice Bubbles™ (Kellogg's, Australia)	87*	30 g	26	22
Rice Chex™ (Nabisco, Canada)	89	30 g	26	23
Rice Krispies™ (Kellogg's, Canada)	82	30 g	26	22
Shredded Wheat (Canada)	67	30 g	20	13
Shredded Wheat™ (Nabisco, Canada)	83	30 g	20	17
Average of two studies	75	30 g	20	15
Special K™ (Kellogg's, Australia)	54	30 g	21	11
Special K™ (Kellogg's, USA)	69	30 g	21	14
Special K™ (Kellogg's, France)	84	30 g	24	20
Soy Tasty™ (Sanitarium, Australia)	60	30 g	20	12
Soytana™ (Vogel's, Australia)	49	45 g	25	12
Sultana Bran™ (Kellogg's, Australia)	73	30 g	19	14
Sustain™ (Kellogg's, Australia)	68	30 g	22	15
Team™ (Nabisco, Canada)	82	30 g	22	17
Thank Goodness™ (Hubbards, New Zealand)	65	30 g	23	15

* Average

FOOD	GI	NOMINAL SERVE SIZE	AVAILABLE CARB PER SERVE	GL PER SERVE
Total™ (General Mills, Canada)	76	30 g	22	17
Ultra-bran™ (Vogel's, Australia)	41	30 g	13	5
Wheat-bites™ (Uncle Toby's, Australia)	72	30 g	25	18
Whole wheat Goldies™ (Kellogg's, Australia)	70	30 g	20	14
Good Start™, muesli wheat biscuits (Sanitarium, Australia)	68	30 g	20	14
Hi-Bran Weet-Bix™, wheat biscuits (Sanitarium, Australia)	61	30 g	17	10
Hi-Bran Weet-Bix™ with soy and linseed (Sanitarium, Australia)	57	30 g	16	9
Honey Goldies™ (Kellogg's Australia)	72	30 g	21	15
Lite-Bix™, plain, no added sugar (Sanitarium, Australia)	70	30 g	20	14
Oat bran Weet-Bix™ (Sanitarium, Australia)	57	30 g	20	11
Sultana Goldies™ (Kellogg's Australia)	65	30 g	21	13

BREAKFAST CEREAL BARS

FOOD	GI	NOMINAL SERVE SIZE	AVAILABLE CARB PER SERVE	GL PER SERVE
Crunchy Nut Cornflakes™ bar (Kellogg's, Australia)	72	30 g	26	19
Fibre Plus™ bar (Uncle Toby's, Australia)	78	30 g	23	18
Fruity-Bix™ bar, fruit and nut (Sanitarium, Australia)	56	30 g	19	10
Fruity-Bix™ bar, wild berry (Sanitarium, Australia)	51	30 g	19	9
K-Time Just Right™ bar (Kellogg's, Australia)	72	30 g	24	17

* Average

FOOD	GI	NOMINAL SERVE SIZE	AVAILABLE CARB PER SERVE	GL PER SERVE
K-Time Strawberry Crunch™ bar (Kellogg's, Australia)	77	30 g	25	19
Rice Bubble Treat™ bar (Kellogg's, Australia)	63	30 g	24	15
Sustain™ bar (Kellogg's, Australia)	57	30 g	25	14

CEREAL GRAINS

Amaranth popped, with milk	97	30 g	22	21

Barley

Barley, pearled (Canada)	22			
Barley (Canada)	22			
Barley, pot, boiled 20 min	25			
Barley (Canada)	27			
Barley, pearled (Canada)	29			
Average of five studies	25	150 g	32	8
Barley, cracked (Malthouth, Tunisia)	50	150 g	42	21
Barley, rolled cooked, dry (Australia)	66	50 g	38	25

Buckwheat

Buckwheat (Canada)	54*	150 g	30	16
Buckwheat groats, boiled 12 min (Sweden)	45	150 g	30	13

Corn/Maize

Maize (Zea mays), flour made into chapatti (India)	59			
Maize meal porridge/gruel (Kenya)	109			

Cornmeal

Cornmeal, boiled in salted water 2 min (Canada)	68	150 g	13	9
Cornmeal with margarine (Canada)	69	150 g	12	9
Average of two studies	69	150 g	13	9

---

* Average

FOOD	GI	NOMINAL SERVE SIZE	AVAILABLE CARB PER SERVE	GL PER SERVE
Corn, sweet				
Corn, sweet, 'Honey & Pearl' variety boiled (New Zealand)	37	150 g	30	11
Corn, sweet, on the cob, boiled 20 min (Australia)	48	150 g	30	14
Corn, sweet, (Canada)	59	150 g	33	20
Corn, sweet, (USA)	60	150 g	33	20
Corn, sweet, (South Africa)	62	150 g	33	20
Average of three studies	53	150 g	32	17
Sweet corn, canned, diet-pack (USA)	46	150 g	28	13
Sweet corn, frozen, reheated in microwave (Canada)	47	150 g	33	16
Taco shells, cornmeal-based, baked (Old El Paso, Canada)	68	20 g	12	8
Couscous				
Couscous, boiled 5 min (USA)	61			
Couscous, boiled 5 min (Tunisia)	69			
Average of two studies	65	150 g	35	23
Millet				
Millet, boiled (Canada)	71	150 g	36	25
Rice, white				
Arborio, risotto rice, boiled (Sun Rice, Australia)	69	150 g	43	29
White (*Oryza sativa*), boiled (India)	69	150 g	43	30
Rice, boiled white				
Type NS (France)	45*	150 g	30	14
Type NS (India)	48	150 g	38	18
Type NS (France)	52	150 g	36	19
Type NS (Pakistan)	69	150 g	38	26

* Average

FOOD	GI	NOMINAL SERVE SIZE	AVAILABLE CARB PER SERVE	GL PER SERVE
Type NS (Canada)	60*	150 g	42	25
Type NS, boiled in salted water (India)	72	150 g	38	27
Type NS, boiled 13 min (Italy)	102	150 g	30	31
Type NS (Kenya)	112	150 g	42	47
Type NS, boiled in salted water, refrigerated 16–20h, reheated (India)	53	150 g	38	20
Type NS, boiled 13 min, then baked 10 min (Italy)	104	150 g	30	31
Rice, Long grain, boiled				
Long grain, boiled 5 min (Canada)	41	150 g	40	16
Long grain, boiled 15 min (Mahatma, Australia)	50	150 g	43	21
Long grain (Uncle Bens®, New Zealand)	56	150 g	43	24
Long grain, boiled 25 min (Surinam)	56	150 g	43	24
Long grain, boiled 15 min	58	150 g	40	23
Gem long grain (Dainty, Canada)	58*	150 g	40	23
Long grain, boiled 7 min (Star, Canada)	64	150 g	40	26
Average of seven studies	55	150 g	41	23
Rice, long grain, quick-cooking varieties				
Long grain, parboiled 10 min cooking time (Uncle Ben's, Belgium)	68	150 g	37	25
Long grain, parboiled, 20 min cooking time (Uncle Ben's, Belgium)	75	150 g	37	28
Long grain, microwaved 2 min (Express Rice, Masterfoods, UK)	52	150 g	37	19

* Average

FOOD	GI	NOMINAL SERVE SIZE	AVAILABLE CARB PER SERVE	GL PER SERVE
Rice, specialty rices				
Cajun Style, Uncle Ben's® (Effem Foods, Canada)	51	150 g	37	19
Garden Style, Uncle Ben's® (Effem Foods, Canada)	55	150 g	37	21
Long Grain and Wild, Uncle Ben's® (Effem Foods, Canada)	54	150 g	37	20
Mexican Fast and Fancy, Uncle Ben's® (Effem Foods, Canada)	58	150 g	37	22
Saskatchewan wild rice (Canada)	57	150 g	32	18
Broken rice, white (Lion Foods, Thailand)	86	150 g	43	37
Glutinous rice, white (Thailand)	98	150 g	32	31
Jasmine rice, white, long grain (Thailand)	109	150 g	42	46
Rice, white low-amylose				
Calrose, white, medium grain, boiled (Rice Growers, Australia)	83	150 g	42	35
Sungold, Pelde, parboiled (Rice Growers, Australia)	87	150 g	43	37
Waxy (0–2% amylose) (Rice Growers, Australia)	88	150 g	43	38
Pelde, white (Rice Growers, Australia)	93	150 g	43	40
White, low-amylose, boiled (Turkey)	139	150 g	43	60
Rice, white high-amylose				
Bangladeshi rice variety BR16 (28% amylose)	37	150 g	39	14
Bangladeshi rice variety BR16, long-grain (27% amylose)	39	150 g	39	15
Average of two studies	38	150 g	39	15

* Average

FOOD	GI	NOMINAL SERVE SIZE	AVAILABLE CARB PER SERVE	GL PER SERVE
Doongara, white (Rice Growers, Australia)	56*	150 g	42	24
Koshikari (Japonica), short-grain, (Japan)	48	150 g	42	20
Rice, Basmati				
Basmati, boiled (Mahatma, Australia)	58	150 g	42	24
Precooked basmati rice, Uncle Ben's Express® (UK)	57	150 g	41	24
Quick-cooking basmati, Uncle Ben's® Superior (Belgium)	60	150 g	38	23
Rice, brown				
Brown (Canada)	66	150 g	33	21
Brown, steamed (USA)	50	150 g	33	16
Brown (Oriza Sativa), boiled (South India)	50	150 g	33	16
Average of three studies	55	150 g	33	18
Calrose brown (Rice Growers, Australia)	87	150 g	40	35
Doongara brown, high-amylose (Rice Growers, Australia)	66	150 g	37	24
Pelde brown (Rice Growers, Australia)	76	150 g	38	29
Parboiled, cooked 20 min, Uncle Ben's Natur-reis ® (Belgium)	64	150 g	36	23
Sunbrown Quick™ (Rice Growers, Australia)	80	150 g	38	31
Rice Instant/puffed				
Instant rice, white, boiled 1 min (Canada)	46	150 g	42	19
Instant rice, white, cooked 6 min (Trice brand, Australia)	87	150 g	42	36

* Average

FOOD	GI	NOMINAL SERVE SIZE	AVAILABLE CARB PER SERVE	GL PER SERVE
Puffed, white, cooked 5 min, Uncle Ben's Snabbris® (Belgium)	74	150 g	42	31
Average of three studies	69	150 g	42	29
Instant Doongara, white, cooked 5 min (Rice Growers, Australia)	94	150 g	42	35
Rice parboiled				
Parboiled rice (Canada)	48	150 g	36	18
Parboiled rice (USA)	72	150 g	36	26
Converted, white, Uncle Ben's® (Canada)	45	150 g	36	16
Converted, white, boiled 20–30 min, Uncle Ben's® (USA)	38	150 g	36	14
Converted, white, long grain, boiled 20–30 min, Uncle Ben's® (USA)	50	150 g	36	18
Boiled, 12 min (Denmark)	43	150 g	36	15
Long grain, boiled 5 min (Canada)	38	150 g	36	14
Long grain, boiled, 10 min (USA)	61	150 g	36	22
Long grain, boiled 15 min (Canada)	47	150 g	36	17
Long grain, boiled 25 min (Canada)	46	150 g	36	17
Average of four studies	49	150 g	36	18
Rice parboiled, low-amylose				
Bangladeshi rice variety BR2, parboiled (12% amylose)	51	150 g	38	19
Parboiled, Sungold (Rice Growers, Australia)	87	150 g	39	34
Rice parboiled, high-amylose				
Parboiled, high-amylose (28%), Doongara (Rice Growers, Australia)	50	150 g	42	21
Bangladeshi rice variety BR16 (28% amylose)	35	150 g	37	13

* Average

FOOD	GI	NOMINAL SERVE SIZE	AVAILABLE CARB PER SERVE	GL PER SERVE
Bangladeshi rice variety BR16, traditional method (27% amylose)	32	150 g	38	12
Bangladeshi rice variety BR16, pressure parboiled (27% amylose)	27	150 g	41	11
Bangladeshi rice variety BR4 (27% amylose)	33	150 g	38	13
Average	35	150 g	39	14
Rye, whole kernels				
Rye, whole kernels, dry (Canada)	29	50 g	38	11
Average of three studies	34	50 g	38	13
Wheat				
Wheat, whole kernels				
Wheat, whole kernels, dry (Triticum aestivum) (India)	30	50 g	38	11
Wheat, whole kernels, dry (Canada)	42	50 g	33	14
Wheat, whole kernels, pressure cooked, dry (Canada)	44	50 g	33	14
Wheat, whole kernels, dry (Canada)	48	50 g	33	16
Average of four studies	41	50 g	34	14
Wheat, type NS, dry (India)	90	50 g	38	34
Wheat, precooked kernels				
Durum wheat, precooked, cooked 20 min, dry (France)	52	50 g	37	19
Durum wheat, precooked, cooked 10 min, dry (France)	50	50 g	33	17
Durum wheat, precooked in pouch, reheated (France)	40	125 g	39	16
Quick-cooking (White Wings, Australia)	54	150 g	47	25

---

* Average

FOOD	GI	NOMINAL SERVE SIZE	AVAILABLE CARB PER SERVE	GL PER SERVE
Semolina				
Semolina, roasted at 105°C then gelatinised with water (India)	55			
Semolina, steamed and gelatinised (India)	54			
Average of two studies	55	150 g	11	6
Wheat cracked (bulghur)				
Bulghur, boiled	47	150 g	26	12

COOKIES

FOOD	GI	NOMINAL SERVE SIZE	AVAILABLE CARB PER SERVE	GL PER SERVE
Arrowroot (McCormicks's, Canada)	63	25 g	20	13
Arrowroot plus (McCormicks's, Canada)	62	25 g	18	11
Milk Arrowroot™ (Arnotts, Australia)	69	25 g	18	12
Average of three studies	65	25 g	19	12
Barquette Abricot (LU, France)	71	40 g	32	23
Bebe Dobre Rano Chocolate (LU, Czech Republic)	57	50 g	33	19
Bebe Dobre Rano Honey and Hazelnuts (LU, Czech Republic)	51	50 g	34	17
Bebe Jemne Susenky (LU, Czech Republic)	67	25 g	20	14
Digestives	59	25 g	16	10
Digestives, gluten-free (Nutricia, UK)	58	25 g	17	10
Evergreen met Krenten (LU, Netherlands)	66	38 g	21	14
Golden Fruit (Griffin's, New Zealand)	77	25 g	17	13
Graham Wafers (Christie Brown, Canada)	74	25 g	18	14

* Average

FOOD	GI	NOMINAL SERVE SIZE	AVAILABLE CARB PER SERVE	GL PER SERVE
Gran'Dia Banana, Oats and Honey (LU, Brazil)	28	30 g	23	6
Grany en-cas Abricot (LU, France)	55	30 g	16	9
Grany en-cas Fruits des bois (LU, France)	50	30 g	14	7
Grany Rush Apricot (LU, Netherlands)	62	30 g	20	12
Highland Oatmeal™ (Westons, Australia)	55	25 g	18	10
Highland Oatcakes (Walker's, Scotland)	57	25 g	15	8
LU P'tit Déjeuner Chocolat (LU, France)	42	50 g	34	14
LU P'tit Déjeuner Miel et Pépites Chocolat (LU, France)	49*	50 g	35	17
Maltmeal wafer (Griffin's, New Zealand)	50	25 g	17	9
Morning Coffee™ (Arnotts, Australia)	79	25 g	19	15
Nutrigrain Fruits des bois (Kellogg's, France)	57	35 g	23	13
Oatmeal (Canada)	54	25 g	17	9
Oro (Saiwa, Italy)	64*	40 g	32	20
Petit LU Normand (LU, France)	51	25 g	19	10
Petit LU Roussillon (LU, France)	48	25 g	18	9
Prince Energie+ (LU, France)	73	25 g	17	13
Prince fourré chocolat (LU, France)	52*	65 g	30	16
Prince Meganana Chocolate (LU, Spain)	49	50 g	36	18
Prince Petit Déjeuner Vanille (LU, France and Spain)	45	50 g	36	16

* Average

FOOD	GI	NOMINAL SERVE SIZE	AVAILABLE CARB PER SERVE	GL PER SERVE
Rich Tea (Canada)	55	25 g	19	10
Sablé des Flandres (LU, France)	57	20 g	15	8
Shortbread (Arnotts, Australia)	64	25 g	16	10
Shredded Wheatmeal™ (Arnotts, Australia)	62	25 g	18	11
Snack Right Fruit Slice (97% fat-free) (Arnott's, Australia)	48	25 g	19	9
Thé (France)	41	20 g	16	6
Vanilla Wafers (Christie Brown, Canada)	77	25 g	18	14
Véritable Petit Beurre (LU, France)	51	25 g	18	9

CRACKERS

FOOD	GI	NOMINAL SERVE SIZE	AVAILABLE CARB PER SERVE	GL PER SERVE
Breton wheat crackers (Dare Foods, Canada)	67	25 g	14	10
Corn Thins, puffed corn cakes, gluten-free (Real Foods, Australia)	87	25 g	20	18
Cream Cracker (LU, Brazil)	65	25 g	17	11
High-calcium cracker (Danone, Malaysia)	52	25 g	17	9
Jatz™, plain salted cracker biscuits (Arnotts, Australia)	55	25 g	17	10
Puffed Crispbread (Westons, Australia)	81	25 g	19	15
Puffed rice cakes (Rice Growers, Australia)	82	25 g	21	17
Rye crispbread (Canada)	63	25 g	16	10
Ryvita™ (Canada)	69	25 g	16	11
High-fibre rye crispbread (Ryvita, UK)	59	25 g	15	9
Rye crispbread (Ryvita, UK)	63	25 g	18	11

* Average

FOOD	GI	NOMINAL SERVE SIZE	AVAILABLE CARB PER SERVE	GL PER SERVE
Average of four studies	64	25 g	16	11
Kavli™ Norwegian Crispbread (Players, Australia)	71	25 g	16	12
Sao™, plain square crackers (Arnotts, Australia)	70	25 g	17	12
Stoned Wheat Thins (Christie Brown, Canada)	67	25 g	17	12
Water cracker (Canada)	63	25 g	18	11
Water cracker (Arnotts, Australia)	78	25 g	18	14
Average of two studies	71	25 g	18	13
Premium Soda Crackers (Christie Brown, Canada)	74	25 g	17	12
Vita-wheat™, original, crispbread (Arnott's, Australia)	55	25 g	19	10

DAIRY PRODUCTS AND ALTERNATIVES

Custard

FOOD	GI	NOMINAL SERVE SIZE	AVAILABLE CARB PER SERVE	GL PER SERVE
No Bake Egg Custard (Nestlé, Australia)	35	100 g	17	6
Custard, home made (Australia)	43	100 g	17	7
TRIM™, reduced-fat custard (Pauls, Australia)	37	100 g	15	6
Average of three studies	38	100 g	16	6

Ice-cream, Regular/NS

FOOD	GI	NOMINAL SERVE SIZE	AVAILABLE CARB PER SERVE	GL PER SERVE
Ice-cream, NS (Canada)	36			
Ice-cream (half vanilla, half chocolate) (Italy)	57			
Ice-cream, NS (USA)	62			
Ice-cream, chocolate flavored (USA)	68			
Ice-cream (half vanilla, half chocolate) (Italy)	80			

* Average

FOOD	GI	NOMINAL SERVE SIZE	AVAILABLE CARB PER SERVE	GL PER SERVE
Average of five studies	61	50 g	13	8
Ice-cream, reduced or low fat				
Ice-cream, vanilla, (Peter's, Australia)	50	50 g	6	3
Ice-cream, (1.2 % fat), Prestige Light vanilla (Norco, Australia)	47	50 g	10	5
Ice-cream, (1.4% fat), Prestige Light toffee (Norco, Australia)	37	50 g	14	5
Ice-cream, Prestige Golden macadamia (Norco, Australia)	37	50 g	9	3
Ice-cream, premium				
Ice-cream, Ultra chocolate, 15% fat (Sara Lee, Australia)	37	50 g	9	4
Ice-cream, French vanilla, 16% fat (Sara Lee, Australia)	38	50 g	9	3
Milk				
Full-fat (Italy)	11			
Full-fat (3% fat, Sweden)	21			
Full-fat (Italy)	24			
Full-fat (Australia)	31			
Full-fat (Canada)	34			
Full-fat (USA)	40			
Average of five studies	27	250 ml	12	3
Fermented cow's milk (ropy milk, Sweden)	11			
Fermented cow's milk (filmjölk, Sweden)	11			
Average of two foods	11			
Milk, skim (Canada)	32	250 g	13	4
Milk, condensed, sweetened (Nestlé, Australia)	61	50 g	28	17

* Average

FOOD	GI	NOMINAL SERVE SIZE	AVAILABLE CARB PER SERVE	GL PER SERVE
Milk, low fat, chocolate, with aspartame, Lite White™ (Australia)	24	250 g	15	3
Milk, low fat, chocolate, with sugar, Lite White™ (Australia)	34	250 g	26	9
Mousse, reduced-fat, made from mix with water				
Butterscotch, 1.9% fat (Nestlé, Australia)	36	50 g	10	4
Chocolate, 2% fat (Nestlé, Australia)	31	50 g	11	3
French vanilla, 2% fat (Nestlé, Australia)	42	100 ml	6	3
Hazelnut, 2.4% fat (Nestlé, Australia)	36	50 g	10	4
Mango, 1.8% fat (Nestlé, Australia)	33	50 g	11	4
Mixed berry, 2.2% fat (Nestlé, Australia)	36	50 g	10	4
Strawberry, 2.3% fat (Nestlé, Australia)	32	50 g	10	3
Average of six foods	34	50 g	10	4
Pudding				
Instant, chocolate, made from powder and milk (White Wings, Australia)	47	100 g	16	7
Instant, vanilla, made from powder and milk (White Wings, Australia)	40	100 g	16	6
Average of two foods	44	100 g	16	7
Yoghurt				
Yoghurt, type (Canada)	36	200 g	9	3
Yoghurt low fat				
Low fat, fruit, aspartame, Ski™ (Dairy Farmers, Australia)	14	200 g	13	2

* Average

FOOD	GI	NOMINAL SERVE SIZE	AVAILABLE CARB PER SERVE	GL PER SERVE
Low fat, fruit, sugar, Ski™ (Dairy Farmers, Australia)	33	200 g	31	10
Low fat (0.9%), fruit, wild strawberry (Ski d'lite™, Dairy Farmers, Australia)	31	200 g	30	9
Yoghurt diet non-fat, with low-calorie sweeteners (no added sugars)				
Yoghurt, no-fat, French Vanilla, Vaalia, with sugar	40	150 g	27	10
Yoghurt, no-fat, Mango, Vaalia, with sugar	39	150 g	25	10
Yoghurt, no-fat, Wildberry, Vaalia, with sugar	38	150 g	22	8
Yoghurt, no-fat, Strawberry, Vaalia, with sugar	38	150 g	22	8
Diet Vaalia™, vanilla (Pauls, Australia)	23	200 g	13	3
mean of five foods	24	200 g	14	3
Yoghurt reduced-fat				
Reduced-fat, Vaalia™, apricot & mango (Pauls, Australia)	26	200 g	30	8
Reduced-fat, Vaalia™, French vanilla (Pauls, Australia)	26	200 g	10	3
Reduced-fat, Extra-Lite™, strawberry (Pauls, Australia)	28	200 g	33	9
mean of three foods	27	200 g	24	7
Yoghurt drink, reduced-fat, Vaalia™, passionfruit (Pauls, Australia)	38	200 g	29	11
Soy-based dairy product alternatives				
Soy milks (containing maltodextrin)				
Soy milk, full-fat, Original (So Natural, Australia)	44	250 g	17	8

* Average

FOOD	GI	NOMINAL SERVE SIZE	AVAILABLE CARB PER SERVE	GL PER SERVE
Soy milk, full-fat, Calciforte (So Natural, Australia)	36	250 g	18	6
Soy milk, reduced-fat, Light (So Natural, Australia)	44	250 g	17	8
Soy milk drinks				
Soy smoothie drink, banana, 1% fat (So Natural, Australia)	30	250 g	22	7
Soy smoothie drink, chocolate hazelnut, 1% fat (So Natural, Australia)	34	250 g	25	8
mean of two drinks	32	250 g	23	7
Up & Go™, cocoa malt flavour (Sanitarium, Australia)	43	250 g	26	11
Up & Go™, original malt flavour (Sanitarium, Australia)	46	250 g	24	11
Average of two drinks	45	250 g	25	11
Xpress™, chocolate (So Natural, Australia)	39	250 g	34	13
Soy yoghurt				
Soy yoghurt, peach and mango, 2% fat, sugar (So Natural, Australia)	50	200 g	26	13
Tofu-based frozen dessert, chocolate (USA)	115	50 g	9	10

FRUIT AND FRUIT PRODUCTS

Apple, (Denmark)	28	120 g	13	4
Apple, Braeburn (New Zealand)	32	120 g	13	4
Apple, s (Canada)	34	120 g	16	5
Apple, Golden Delicious (Canada)	39	120 g	16	6
Apple, (USA)	40	120 g	16	6

* Average

FOOD	GI	NOMINAL SERVE SIZE	AVAILABLE CARB PER SERVE	GL PER SERVE
Apple, (Italy)	44	120 g	13	6
Average of six studies	38	120 g	15	6
Apple, dried (Australia)	29	60 g	34	10
Apple juice, unsweetened, reconstituted (Berri, Australia)	39	250 g	25	10
Apple juice, unsweetened (USA)	40	250 g	29	12
Apple juice, unsweetened (Allens, Canada)	41	250 g	30	12
Average of three studies	40	250 g	28	11
Apricots, raw (Italy)	57	120 g	9	5
Apricots, canned in light syrup (Riviera, Canada)	64	120 g	19	12
Apricots, dried (Australia)	30	60 g	27	8
Apricots, dried (Wasco, Canada)	32	60 g	30	10
Average of two studies	31	60 g	28	9
Apricot fruit bar, (Mother Earth, New Zealand)	50	50 g	34	17
Apricot fruit spread, (Glen Ewin, Australia)	55	30 g	13	7
Apricot Fruity Bitz™ (Blackmores, Australia)	42	15 g	12	5
Banana (Canada)	46	120 g	25	12
Banana (Italy)	58	120 g	23	13
Banana (Canada)	58	120 g	25	15
Banana (Canada)	62	120 g	25	16
Banana (South Africa)	70	120 g	23	16
Banana, ripe (all yellow) (USA)	51	120 g	25	13
Banana, under-ripe (Denmark)	30	120 g	21	6
Banana, slightly under-ripe (yellow with green sections) (USA)	42	120 g	25	11

* Average

FOOD	GI	NOMINAL SERVE SIZE	AVAILABLE CARB PER SERVE	GL PER SERVE
Banana, over-ripe (yellow flecked with brown) (USA)	48	120 g	25	12
Banana, over-ripe (Denmark)	52	120 g	20	11
Average of 10 studies	52	120 g	24	12
Banana, processed fruit fingers, Heinz Kidz™ (Australia)	61	30 g	20	12
Breadfruit (*Artocarpus altilis*), raw (Australia)	68	120 g	27	18
Cherries, raw, NS[8] (Canada)	22	120 g	12	3
Chico (*Zapota zapotilla coville*), raw (Philippines)	40	120 g	29	12
Cranberry juice cocktail (Ocean Spray, Australia)	52	250 g	31	16
Cranberry juice cocktail (Ocean Spray, USA)	68	250 g	35	24
Cranberry juice drink (Ocean Spray®, UK)	56	250 g	29	16
Custard apple, raw, flesh only (Australia)	54	120 g	19	10
Dates, dried (Australia)	103	60 g	40	42
Figs, dried, tenderised (Dessert Maid, Australia)	61	60 g	26	16
Fruit Cocktail, canned (Delmonte, Canada)	55	120 g	16	9
Grapefruit, raw (Canada)	25	120 g	11	3
Grapefruit juice, unsweetened (Sunpac, Canada)	48	250 g	20	9
Grapes, NS (Canada)	43	120 g	17	7
Grapes, NS (Italy)	49	120 g	19	9
Average of two studies	46	120 g	18	8
Grapes, black, Waltham Cross (Australia)	59	120 g	18	11

* Average

FOOD	GI	NOMINAL SERVE SIZE	AVAILABLE CARB PER SERVE	GL PER SERVE
Kiwi fruit, Hayward (New Zealand)	47	120 g	12	5
Kiwi fruit (Australia)	58	120 g	12	7
Average of two studies	53	120 g	12	6
Lychee, canned in syrup and drained, Narcissus brand (China)	79	120 g	20	16
Mango (*Mangifera indica*) (Philippines)	41	120 g	20	8
Mango (*Mangifera indica*) (Australia)	51	120 g	15	8
Mango, ripe (*Mangifera indica*) (India)	60	120 g	15	9
Average of three studies	51	120 g	17	8
Mango, Frutia™ (Weis, Australia)	42	100 g	23	10
Marmalade, orange (Australia)	48	30 g	20	9
Oranges, NS (Denmark)	31	120 g	11	3
Oranges, NS (South Africa)	33	120 g	10	3
Oranges, NS (Canada)	40	120 g	11	4
Oranges, NS s (Italy)	48	120 g	11	5
Oranges (Sunkist, USA)	48	120 g	11	5
Oranges NS (Canada)	51	120 g	11	6
Average of six studies	42	120 g	11	5
Orange juice (Canada)	46	250 g	26	12
Orange juice, reconstituted (Quelch, Australia)	53	250 g	18	9
Orange juice, reconstituted from frozen concentrate (USA)	57	250 g	26	15
Average of three studies	52	250 g	23	12
Paw paw (Carica papaya) (Australia)	56	120 g	8	5
Paw paw, ripe (India)	60	120 g	29	17
Papaya (*Carica papaya*) (Philippines)	60	120 g	15	9
Average of three studies	59	120 g	17	10
Peach, raw (Canada)	28	120 g	13	4
Peach, raw (Italy)	56	120 g	8	5
Average of two studies	42	120 g	11	5

* Average

FOOD	GI	NOMINAL SERVE SIZE	AVAILABLE CARB PER SERVE	GL PER SERVE
Peach, canned in natural juice (Ardmona, Australia)	30	120 g	11	3
Peach, canned in natural juice (SPC, Australia)	45	120 g	11	5
Average of two studies	38	120 g	11	4
Peach, canned in heavy syrup (Letona, Australia)	58	120 g	15	9
Peach, canned in light syrup (Delmonte, Canada)	52	120 g	18	9
Peach, canned in reduced-sugar syrup (SPC, Australia)	62	120 g	17	11
Pear, raw, NS (Canada)	33	120 g	13	4
Pear, Winter Nellis, raw (New Zealand)	34	120 g	12	4
Pear, Bartlett, raw (Canada)	41	120 g	8	3
Pear, raw NS (Italy)	42	120 g	11	4
Average of four studies	38	120 g	11	4
Pear halves, canned in reduced-sugar syrup, SPC Lite (Australia)	25	120 g	14	4
Pear halves, canned in natural juice (SPC, Australia)	43	120 g	13	5
Pear, canned in pear juice, Bartlett (Delmonte, Canada)	44	120 g	11	5
Pineapple, raw (Australia)	66	120 g	10	6
Pineapple (*Ananas comosus*), raw (Philippines)	51	120 g	16	8
Average of two studies	59	120 g	13	7
Pineapple juice, unsweetened (Dole, Canada)	46	250 g	34	15
Plum, raw, NS (Canada)	24	120 g	14	3
Plum, raw, NS (Italy)	53	120 g	11	6
Average of two studies	39	120 g	12	5

* Average

FOOD	GI	NOMINAL SERVE SIZE	AVAILABLE CARB PER SERVE	GL PER SERVE
Prunes, pitted (Sunsweet, USA)	29	60 g	33	10
Raisins (Canada)	64	60 g	44	28
Rockmelon/Cantaloupe, raw (Australia)	65	120 g	6	4
Strawberries, fresh, raw (Australia)	40	120 g	3	1
Strawberry jam	51	30 g	20	10
Strawberry Real Fruit Bars (Uncle Toby's, Australia)	90	30 g	26	23
Sultanas	56	60 g	45	25
Tomato juice, no added sugar (Berri, Australia)	38	250 g	9	4
Tropical Fruity Bitz™, (Blackmores, Australia)	41	15 g	11	5
Vitari, wild berry, non-dairy, frozen dessert (Nestlé, Australia)	59	100 g	21	12
Watermelon, raw (Australia)	72	120 g	6	4
Wild Berry Fruity Bitz™ (Blackmores, Australia)	35	15 g	12	4

INFANT FORMULA AND WEANING FOODS

Formula

FOOD	GI	NOMINAL SERVE SIZE	AVAILABLE CARB PER SERVE	GL PER SERVE
Infasoy™, soy-based, milk-free (Wyeth, Australia)	55	100 ml	7	4
Karicare™ formula with omega oils (Nutricia, New Zealand)	35	100 ml	7	2
Nan-1™ infant formula with iron (Nestlé, Australia)	30	100 ml	8	2
S-26™ infant formula (Wyeth, Australia)	36	100 ml	7	3

* Average

FOOD	GI	NOMINAL SERVE SIZE	AVAILABLE CARB PER SERVE	GL PER SERVE
Weaning Foods				
Farex™ baby rice (Heinz, Australia)	95	87 g	6	6
Robinsons First Tastes from 4 months (Nutricia, UK)				
Apple, apricot and banana cereal	56	75 g	13	7
Creamed porridge	59	75 g	9	5
Rice pudding	59	75 g	11	6
Heinz for Baby from 4 months (Heinz, Australia)				
Chicken and noodles with vegetables, strained	67	120 g	7	5
Sweetcorn and rice	65	120 g	15	10

LEGUMES AND NUTS

FOOD	GI	NOMINAL SERVE SIZE	AVAILABLE CARB PER SERVE	GL PER SERVE
Baked Beans				
Baked Beans, canned (Canada)	40			
Baked Beans, canned beans in tomato sauce (Libby, Canada)	56			
Average of two studies	48	150 g	17	8
Beans, dried, boiled				
Beans, dried, type NS (Italy)	36	150 g	30	11
Beans, dried, type NS (Italy)	20	150 g	30	6
Average of two studies	29	150 g	30	9
Blackeyed beans/peas (Cowpeas), boiled				
Blackeyed beans (Canada)	50	150 g	21	11
Blackeyed beans (Canada)	33	150 g	21	7
Average of two studies	42	150 g	21	9
Butter Beans				
Butter beans (South Africa)	28	150 g	20	5

* Average

FOOD	GI	NOMINAL SERVE SIZE	AVAILABLE CARB PER SERVE	GL PER SERVE
Butter beans, dried, cooked (South Africa)	29	150 g	20	6
Butter beans (Canada)	36	150 g	20	7
Average of three studies	31	150 g	20	6
Butter beans, dried, boiled + 5g sucrose (South Africa)	30	150 g	20	6
Butter beans, dried, boiled + 10g sucrose (South Africa)	31	150 g	20	6
Butter beans, dried, boiled + 15g sucrose (South Africa)	54	150 g	20	11
Chickpeas (Garbanzo beans, Bengal gram), boiled				
Chickpeas (Cicer arietinum Linn), boiled (Philippines)	10	150 g	24	2
Chickpeas, dried, boiled (Canada)	31	150 g	24	7
Chickpeas (Canada)	35*	150 g	24	8
Average of three studies	25	150 g	24	6
Chickpeas, canned in brine (Lancia-Bravo, Canada)	42	150 g	22	9
Chickpeas, curry, canned (Canasia, Canada)	41	150 g	16	7
Haricot/navy beans				
Haricot/navy beans, pressure cooked (King Grains, Canada)	29	150 g	33	9
Haricot/navy beans, dried, boiled (Canada)	30	150 g	30	9
Haricot/navy beans, boiled (Canada)	31	150 g	30	9
Haricot/navy beans (King Grains, Canada)	39	150 g	30	12
Haricot/navy beans, pressure cooked (King Grains, Canada)	59	150 g	33	19
Average of five studies	38	150 g	31	12

* Average

FOOD	GI	NOMINAL SERVE SIZE	AVAILABLE CARB PER SERVE	GL PER SERVE
Kidney Beans				
Kidney/white bean (Phaseolus vulgaris Linn), boiled (Philippines)	13	150 g	25	3
Kidney beans (Phaseolus vulgaris) (India)	19	150 g	25	5
Kidney beans (USA)	23	150 g	25	6
Kidney beans, dried, boiled (France)	23	150 g	25	6
Kidney beans (*Phaseolus vulgaris* L.), red, boiled (Sweden)	25	150 g	25	6
Kidney beans (Canada)	29	150 g	25	7
Kidney beans, dried, boiled (Canada)	42	150 g	25	10
Kidney beans (Canada)	46	150 g	25	11
mean of eight studies	28	150 g	25	7
Kidney beans (*Phaseolus vulgaris* L.) – autoclaved	34	150 g	25	8
Kidney beans, canned (Lancia-Bravo, Canada)	52	150 g	17	9
Kidney beans, soaked 12 h, stored moist 24 h, steamed 1 h (India)	70	150 g	25	17
Lentils, type NS				
Lentils, type NS (USA)	28			
Lentils, type NS (Canada)	29			
Average of two studies	29	150 g	18	5
Lentils, green				
Lentils, green, dried, boiled (Canada)	22	150 g	18	4
Lentils, green, dried, boiled (France)	30	150 g	18	6
Lentils, green, dried, boiled (Australia)	37	150 g	14	5
Average of three studies	30	150 g	17	5
Lentils, green, canned in brine (Lancia-Bravo Foods Ltd., Canada)	52	150 g	17	9

* Average

FOOD	GI	NOMINAL SERVE SIZE	AVAILABLE CARB PER SERVE	GL PER SERVE
Lentils, red				
Lentils, red, dried, boiled (Canada)	18	150 g	18	3
Lentils, red, dried, boiled (Canada)	21	150 g	18	4
Lentils, red, dried, boiled (Canada)	31	150 g	18	6
Lentils, red, dried, boiled (Canada)	32	150 g	18	6
Average of four studies	26	150 g	18	5
Lima beans				
Lima beans, baby, frozen (York, Canada)	32	150 g	30	10
Marrowfat peas				
Marrowfat peas, dried, boiled (USA)	31			
Marrowfat peas, dried, boiled (Canada)	47			
Average of two studies	39	150 g	19	7
Mung beans				
Mung bean (Phaseolus areus Roxb), boiled (Philippines)	31	150 g	17	5
Mung bean, fried (Australia)	53			
Mung bean, germinated (Australia)	25	150 g	17	4
Mung bean, pressure cooked (Australia)	42	150 g	17	7
Pinto beans				
Pinto beans, boiled (Canada)	39	150 g	26	10
Pinto beans, canned in brine (Lancia-Bravo, Canada)	45	150 g	22	10
Romano beans (Canada)	46	150 g	18	8
Soy beans				
Soy beans, boiled (Canada)	15	150 g	6	1
Soy beans, boiled (Australia)	20	150 g	6	1
Average of two studies	18	150 g	6	1
Soy beans, canned (Canada)	14	150 g	6	1

* Average

FOOD	GI	NOMINAL SERVE SIZE	AVAILABLE CARB PER SERVE	GL PER SERVE

MEAL REPLACEMENT PRODUCTS

FOOD	GI	NOMINAL SERVE SIZE	AVAILABLE CARB PER SERVE	GL PER SERVE
Hazelnut and Apricot bar (Dietworks, Australia)	42	50 g	22	9
L.E.A.N™ products (Usana, USA)				
L.E.A.N Fibergy™ bar, Harvest Oat	45	50 g	29	13
Nutrimeal™, drink powder, Dutch Chocolate	26	250 g	13	3
L.E.A.N (Life long) Nutribar™, Peanut Crunch	30	40 g	19	6
L.E.A.N (Life long) Nutribar™, Chocolate Crunch	32	40 g	19	6
Average of two Nutribars	31	40 g	19	6
Worldwide Sport Nutrition low-carbohydrate products (USA)				
Designer chocolate, sugar-free	14	35 g	22	3
Burn-it™ bars				
Chocolate deluxe	29	50 g	8	2
Peanut butter	23	50 g	6	1
Pure-protein™ bars				
Chewy choc-chip	30	80 g	14	4
Chocolate deluxe	38	80 g	13	5
Peanut butter	22	80 g	9	2
Strawberry shortcake	43	80 g	13	6
White chocolate mousse	40	80 g	15	6
Pure-protein™ cookies				
Choc-chip cookie dough	25	55 g	11	3
Coconut	42	55 g	9	4
Peanut butter	37	55 g	9	3

* Average

FOOD	GI	NOMINAL SERVE SIZE	AVAILABLE CARB PER SERVE	GL PER SERVE

MIXED MEALS AND CONVENIENCE FOODS

FOOD	GI	NOMINAL SERVE SIZE	AVAILABLE CARB PER SERVE	GL PER SERVE
Chicken nuggets, frozen, reheated (Australia)	46	100 g	16	7
Fish Fingers (Canada)	38	100 g	19	7
Fish fillet, reduced fat, crumbed (Maggi)	43	85 g	16	7
Greek lentil stew with a bread roll, home made (Australia)	40	360 g	37	15
Kugel (Polish dish containing egg noodles, sugar, cheese and raisins) (Israel)	65	150 g	48	31
Lean Cuisine™, chicken with rice (Nestlé, Australia)	36	400 g	68	24
Pies, beef, party size (Farmland, Australia)	45	100 g	27	12
Pizza, cheese (Pillsbury, Canada)	60	100 g	27	16
Pizza, plain (Italy)	80	100 g	27	22
Pizza, Super Supreme, pan (Pizza Hut, Australia)	36	100 g	24	9
Pizza, Super Supreme, thin and crispy (Pizza Hut, Australia)	30	100 g	22	7
Pizza, Vegetarian Supreme, thin and crispy (Pizza Hut, Australia)	49	100 g	25	12
Sausages NS (Canada)	28	100 g	3	1
Sirloin chop with mixed vegetables and mashed potato (Australia)	66	360 g	53	35
Spaghetti bolognaise, home made (Australia)	52	360 g	48	25
Stirfried vegetables with chicken and rice, home made (Australia)	73	360 g	75	55

* Average

FOOD	GI	NOMINAL SERVE SIZE	AVAILABLE CARB PER SERVE	GL PER SERVE
Sushi, salmon (Australia)	48	100 g	36	17
Sushi, roasted sea algae, vinegar and rice (Japan)	55	100 g	37	20
Average of two studies	52	100 g	37	19
Tuna pattie, reduced fat (Maggi)	45	84 g	17	8
White boiled rice, grilled beefburger, cheese, and butter (France)	27	440 g	50	14
White boiled rice, grilled beefburger, cheese and butter (France)	22	440 g	50	11
Average in two groups of subjects	25	440 g	50	13
White bread with toppings				
White bread, butter, regular cow's milk cheese and fresh cucumber (Sweden)	55	200 g	68	38
White bread, butter, yoghurt and pickled cucumber (Sweden)	39	200 g	28	11
White bread with butter (Canada)	59	100 g	48	29
White bread with skim milk cheese (Canada)	55	100 g	47	26
White bread with butter and skim milk cheese (Canada)	62	100 g	38	23
White/wholemeal bread with peanut butter (Canada)	51	100 g	44	23
White/wholemeal bread with peanut butter (Canada)	67	100 g	44	30
Average of two studies	59	100 g	44	26

NUTS

Cashew nuts, salted (Coles Supermarkets, Australia)	22	50 g	13	3
Pecans, raw	10	50 g	3	0
Peanuts, crushed (South Africa)	7	50 g	4	0

* Average

FOOD	GI	NOMINAL SERVE SIZE	AVAILABLE CARB PER SERVE	GL PER SERVE
Peanuts (Canada)	13	50 g	7	1
Peanuts (Mexico)	23	50 g	7	2
Average of three studies	14	50 g	6	1

NUTRITIONAL SUPPORT PRODUCTS

FOOD	GI	NOMINAL SERVE SIZE	AVAILABLE CARB PER SERVE	GL PER SERVE
Choice dm™, vanilla (Mead Johnson, USA)	23	237 ml	24	6
Enercal Plus™ (Wyeth-Ayerst, USA)	61	237 ml	40	24
Enrich Plus™ shake, vanilla	58	200 ml	40	23
Ensure™ (Abbott, Australia)	50	237 ml	40	19
Ensure™, vanilla (Abbott, Australia)	48	250 ml	34	16
Ensure™ bar, chocolate fudge brownie (Abbott, Australia)	43	38 g	20	8
Ensure Plus™, vanilla (Abbott, Australia)	40	237 ml	47	19
Ensure Pudding™, vanilla (Abbott, USA)	36	113 g	26	9
Glucerna™ bar, lemon crunch	27	38 g	20	5
Glucerna™ SR shake, vanilla	19	230 ml	24	5
Glucerna™, vanilla (Abbott, USA)	31	237 ml	23	7
Jevity™ (Abbott, Australia)	48	237 ml	36	17
Resource Diabetic™, vanilla (Novartis, USA)	34	237 ml	23	8
Resource Diabetic™, chocolate (Novartis, New Zealand)	16	237 ml	41	7
Resource™ thickened orange juice (Novartis, New Zealand)	47	237 ml	39	18
Resource™ thickened orange juice (Novartis, New Zealand)	54	237 ml	36	19
Resource™ fruit beverage, peach flavour (Novartis, New Zealand)	40	237 ml	41	16

* Average

FOOD	GI	NOMINAL SERVE SIZE	AVAILABLE CARB PER SERVE	GL PER SERVE
Resource Plus, chocolate	43	237 ml	52	22
Sustagen™, Dutch Chocolate (Mead Johnson, Australia)	31	250 ml	41	13
Sustagen™ Hospital with extra fibre (Mead Johnson, Australia)	33	250 ml	44	15
Sustagen™ Instant Pudding, vanilla (Mead Johnson, Australia)	27	250 g	47	13
Ultracal™ with fiber (Mead Johnson, USA)	40	237 ml	29	12

PASTA and NOODLES

FOOD	GI	NOMINAL SERVE SIZE	AVAILABLE CARB PER SERVE	GL PER SERVE
Capellini (Primo, Canada)	45	180 g	45	20
Corn pasta, gluten-free (Orgran, Australia)	78	180 g	42	32
Fettucine, egg				
Fettucine, egg	32	180 g	46	15
Fettucine, egg (Mother Earth, Australia)	47	180 g	46	22
Average of two studies	40	180 g	46	18
Gnocchi				
Gnocchi, NS (Latina, Australia)	68	180 g	48	33
Instant noodles				
Instant 'two-minute' noodles, Maggi® (Australia)	46			
Instant 'two-minute' noodles, Maggi® (New Zealand)	48			
Instant noodles (Mr Noodle, Canada)	47			
Average of three studies	47	180 g	40	19

* Average

FOOD	GI	NOMINAL SERVE SIZE	AVAILABLE CARB PER SERVE	GL PER SERVE
Linguine				
Thick, durum wheat, white, fresh (Sweden)	43	180 g	48	21
Thick, fresh, durum wheat flour (Sweden)	48	180 g	48	23
Average of two studies	46	180 g	48	22
Thin, durum wheat (Sweden)	49	180 g	48	23
Thin, fresh, durum wheat flour (Sweden)	61	180 g	48	29
Average of four studies	52	180 g	45	23
Mung bean noodles				
Lungkow beanthread noodles (National Cereals, China)	26	180 g	45	12
Mung bean noodles (Longkou beanthread) (Yantai, China)	39	180 g	45	18
Average of two studies	33			
Macaroni				
Macaroni, plain, boiled 5 min (Lancia-Bravo, Canada)	45	180 g	49	22
Macaroni, plain, boiled (Turkey)	48	180 g	49	23
Average of two studies	47	180 g	48	23
Macaroni and Cheese, boxed (Kraft, Canada)	64	180 g	51	32
Ravioli				
Ravioli (Australia)	39	180 g	38	15
Rice noodles/pasta				
Rice noodles, dried, boiled (Thai World, Thailand)	61	180 g	39	23
Rice noodles, freshly made, boiled (Sydney, Australia)	40	180 g	39	15

* Average

FOOD	GI	NOMINAL SERVE SIZE	AVAILABLE CARB PER SERVE	GL PER SERVE
Rice pasta, brown, boiled 16 min (Rice Growers, Australia)	92	180 g	38	35
Rice and maize pasta, gluten-free, Ris'O'Mais (Orgran, Australia)	76	180 g	49	37
Rice vermicelli, Kongmoon (China)	58	180 g	39	22
Spaghetti				
Spaghetti, gluten-free, canned in tomato sauce (Orgran, Australia)	68	220 g	27	19
Spaghetti, protein enriched, boiled 7 min (Catelli, Canada)	27	180 g	52	14
Spaghetti, white, boiled 5 min				
Boiled 5 min (Lancia-Bravo, Canada)	32	180 g	48	15
Boiled 5 min (Canada)	37*	180 g	48	18
Boiled 5 min (Middle East)	44	180 g	48	21
Average of three studies	38	180 g	48	18
Spaghetti, white or type NS, boiled 10-15 min				
White, durum wheat, boiled 10 min (Barilla, Italy)	58	180 g	48	28
White, durum wheat flour, boiled 12 min (Starhushålls, Sweden)	47	180 g	48	23
White, durum wheat flour, boiled 12 min (Sweden)	53	180 g	48	25
Boiled 15 min (Lancia-Bravo, Canada)	32	180 g	48	15
Boiled 15 min (Lancia-Bravo, Canada)				
Boiled 15 min (Canada)	41	180 g	48	20
White, boiled 15 min in salted water (Unico, Canada)	44	180 g	48	21
Average of seven studies	44	180 g	48	21

* Average

FOOD	GI	NOMINAL SERVE SIZE	AVAILABLE CARB PER SERVE	GL PER SERVE
Spaghetti, white or type NS, boiled 20 min				
White, durum wheat, boiled 20 min (Australia)	58	180 g	44	26
Durum wheat, boiled 20 min (USA)	64	180 g	43	27
Average of two studies	61	180 g	44	27
Spaghetti, white, boiled				
White (Denmark)	33	180 g	48	16
White, durum wheat (Catelli, Canada)	34	180 g	48	16
White (Australia)	38	180 g	44	17
White (Canada)	47*	180 g	48	23
White (Vetta, Australia)	49	180 g	44	22
Average of five studies	42	180 g	47	20
Spaghetti, white, durum wheat semolina (Panzani, France)				
Boiled for 11 min	59	180 g	48	28
Boiled for 16.5 min	65	180 g	48	31
Boiled for 22 min	46	180 g	48	22
Average of three cooking times	57	180 g	48	27
Spaghetti, wholemeal, boiled				
Wholemeal (USA)	32	180 g	44	14
Wholemeal (Canada)	42	180 g	40	17
Average of two studies	37	180 g	42	16
Spirali				
Spirali, durum wheat, white, boiled (Vetta, Australia)	43	180 g	44	19
Tortellini				
Tortellini, cheese (Stouffer, Canada)	50	180 g	21	10
Udon noodles				

* Average

FOOD	GI	NOMINAL SERVE SIZE	AVAILABLE CARB PER SERVE	GL PER SERVE
Udon noodles, plain, reheated 5 min (Australia)	62	180 g	48	30
Vermicelli				
Vermicelli, white, boiled (Australia)	35	180 g	44	16

PROTEIN FOODS

Beef	[0]	120 g	0	0
Cheese	[0]	120 g	0	0
Eggs	[0]	120 g	0	0
Fish	[0]	120 g	0	0
Lamb	[0]	120 g	0	0
Pork	[0]	120 g	0	0
Salami	[0]	120 g	0	0
Shellfish (prawns, crab, lobster etc)	[0]	120 g	0	0
Tuna	[0]	120 g	0	0
Veal	[0]	120 g	0	0

SNACK FOODS AND CONFECTIONERY

Burger Rings™ (Smith's, Australia)	90	50 g	31	28
Chocolate, milk, plain with sucrose (Belgium)	34	50 g	22	7
Chocolate, milk (Cadbury's, Australia)	49	50 g	30	14
Chocolate, milk, Dove® (Mars, Australia)	45	50 g	30	13
Chocolate, milk (Nestlé, Australia)	42	50 g	31	13
Average of four studies	43	50 g	28	12
Chocolate, milk, plain, low-sugar with maltitol (Belgium)	35	50 g	22	8
Chocolate, white, Milky Bar® (Nestlé, Australia)	44	50 g	29	13

* Average

FOOD	GI	NOMINAL SERVE SIZE	AVAILABLE CARB PER SERVE	GL PER SERVE
Corn chips, plain, salted (Doritos™, Australia)	42	50 g	25	11
Corn chips, Nachips™ (Old El Paso, Canada)	74	50 g	29	21
Average of three studies	63	50 g	26	17
Fruit bar apricot filled (Mother Earth, New Zealand)	50	50 g	34	17
Fruit Fingers Heinz Kidz™, banana (Heinz, Australia)	61	30 g	20	12
Fruity Bitz™, apricot (Blackmores, Australia)	42	15 g	12	5
Fruity Bitz™, berry (Blackmores, Australia)	35	15 g	12	4
Fruity Bitz™, tropical (Blackmores, Australia)	41	15 g	11	5
Average of three flavours	39	15 g	12	4
Jelly beans, assorted colors (Australia)	78*	30 g	28	22
Kudos Whole Grain Bars, chocolate chip (USA)	62	50 g	32	20
Life Savers®, peppermint candy (Nestlé, Australia)	70	30 g	30	21
M & M's®, peanut (Australia)	33	30 g	17	6
Mars Bar® (Australia)	62	60 g	40	25
Mars Bar® (USA)	68	60 g	40	27
Average of two studies	65	60 g	40	26
Muesli bar containing dried fruit (Uncle Toby's, Australia)	61	30 g	21	13
Nougat, Jijona (La Fama, Spain)	32	30 g	12	4
Nutella®, chocolate hazelnut spread (Australia)	33	20 g	12	4

* Average

FOOD	GI	NOMINAL SERVE SIZE	AVAILABLE CARB PER SERVE	GL PER SERVE
Nuts, cashew salted (Coles Supermarkets, Australia)	22	50 g	13	3
Peanuts, crushed (South Africa)	7	50 g	4	0
Peanuts (Canada)	13	50 g	7	1
Peanuts (Mexico)	23	50 g	7	2
Average of three studies	14	50 g	6	1
Pecan				
Popcorn, plain, cooked in microwave oven (Green's, Australia)	55	20 g	11	6
Popcorn, plain, cooked in microwave oven (Uncle Toby's, Australia)	89	20 g	11	10
Average of two studies	72	20 g	11	8
Pop Tarts™, double choc (Kellogg's, Australia)	70	50 g	35	24
Potato crisps, plain, salted (Arnott's, Australia)	57	50 g	18	10
Potato crisps, plain, salted (Canada)	51	50 g	24	12
Average of two studies	54	50 g	21	11
Pretzels, (Parker's, Australia)	83	30 g	20	16
Real Fruit Bars, strawberry (Uncle Toby's, Australia)	90	30 g	26	23
Roll-Ups® (Uncle Toby's, Australia)	99	30 g	25	24
Skittles® (Australia)	70	50 g	45	32
Snack bar, Apple Cinnamon (Con Agra, USA)	40	50 g	29	12
Snack bar, Peanut Butter & Choc-Chip (USA)	37	50 g	27	10
Snickers Bar® (Australia)	41	60 g	36	15
Snickers Bar® (USA)	68	60 g	34	23
Average of two studies	55	60 g	35	19
Sunripe school straps	40	15 g	11	4
Twisties™ cheese (Smith's, Australia)	74	50 g	29	22

* Average

FOOD	GI	NOMINAL SERVE SIZE	AVAILABLE CARB PER SERVE	GL PER SERVE
Twix® Cookie Bar, caramel (USA)	44	60 g	39	17
SPORTS BARS				
Power Bar®, chocolate (USA)	56*	65 g	42	24
Ironman PR bar®, chocolate (USA)	39	65 g	26	10
SOUPS				
Black Bean (Wil-Pack, USA)	64	250 ml	27	17
Green Pea, canned (Campbell's, Canada)	66	250 ml	41	27
Lentil, canned (Unico, Canada)	44	250 ml	21	9
Minestrone, Country Ladle™ (Campbell's, Australia)	39	250 ml	18	7
Noodle soup (Turkish soup with stock and noodles)	1	250 ml	9	0
Split Pea (Wil-Pak, USA)	60	250 ml	27	16
Tarhana soup (Turkish soup)	20			
Tomato soup (Canada)	38	250 ml	17	6
SUGARS				
Blue Agave cactus nectar, high-fructose				
Organic Agave Cactus Nectar, light, 90% fructose (Western Commerce, USA)	11	10 g	8	1
Organic Agave Cactus Nectar, light, 97% fructose (Western Commerce, USA)	10	10 g	8	1
Fructose				
25g portion (Canada)	11			
50g portion (Canada)	12			
50g portion	20			

* Average

FOOD	GI	NOMINAL SERVE SIZE	AVAILABLE CARB PER SERVE	GL PER SERVE
50g portion	21			
50g portion (USA)	24			
25g portion, fed with oats	25			
Average of six studies	19	10 g	10	2
Glucose				
Dextrose	100	10 g	10	10
Glucose consumed with 3 g American ginseng	78	10 g	10	8
Glucose consumed with gum/fibre				
15 g apple and orange fibre (FITA, Australia)	79	10 g	8	6
14.5 g guar gum	62	10 g	10	6
14.5 g oat gum (78% oat ß-glucan)	57	10 g	10	6
20 g acacia gum	85	10 g	10	9
Honey				
Locust honey (Romania)	32	25 g	21	7
Yellow box (Australia)	35	25 g	18	6
Stringy Bark (Australia)	44	25 g	21	9
Red Gum (Australia)	46	25 g	18	8
Iron Bark (Australia)	48	25 g	15	7
Yapunya (Australia)	52	25 g	17	9
Pure (Capilano, Australia)	58	25 g	21	12
Commercial Blend (Australia)	62	25 g	18	11
Salvation Jane (Australia)	64	25 g	15	10
Commercial Blend (Australia)	72	25 g	13	9
Honey NS (Canada)	87	25 g	21	18
Average of 11 types of honey	55	25 g	18	10
Lactose				
Lactose	46	10 g	10	5
Maltose				
Maltose	105	10 g	10	11

* Average

FOOD	GI	NOMINAL SERVE SIZE	AVAILABLE CARB PER SERVE	GL PER SERVE
Sucrose				
Sucrose	61	10 g	10	6

VEGETABLES

FOOD	GI	NOMINAL SERVE SIZE	AVAILABLE CARB PER SERVE	GL PER SERVE
Artichokes	[0]	80 g	0	0
Avocado	[0]	80 g	0	0
Beetroot	64	80 g	7	5
Bokchoy	[0]	80 g	0	0
Broad beans	79	80 g	11	9
Broccoli	[0]	80 g	0	0
Cabbage	[0]	80 g	0	0
Carrots, peeled, boiled (Australia)	49	80 g	5	2
Cassava, boiled, with salt (Kenya, Africa)	46	100 g	27	12
Capsicum	[0]	80 g	0	0
Cauliflower	[0]	80 g	0	0
Celery	[0]	80 g	0	0
Corn, sweet, 'Honey & Pearl' variety (New Zealand)	37	80 g	16	6
Corn, sweet, on the cob, boiled (Australia)	48	80 g	16	8
Corn, sweet, (Canada)	59	80 g	18	11
Corn, sweet, boiled (USA)	60	80 g	18	11
Corn, sweet, (South Africa)	62	80 g	18	11
Average of five studies	54	80 g	17	9
Corn, sweet, diet-pack, (USA)	46	80 g	14	7
Corn, sweet, frozen (Canada)	47	80 g	15	7
Cucumber	[0]	80 g	0	0
French beans (runner beans)	[0]	80 g	0	0
Leafy vegetables (spinach, rocket etc)	[0]	80 g	0	0
Lettuce	[0]	80 g	0	0

* Average

FOOD	GI	NOMINAL SERVE SIZE	AVAILABLE CARB PER SERVE	GL PER SERVE
Parsnips	97	80 g	12	12
Peas, frozen, boiled (Canada)	39	80 g	7	3
Peas, frozen, boiled (Canada)	51	80 g	7	4
Peas, green (*Pisum sativum*) (India)	54	80 g	7	4
Average of three studies	48	80 g	7	3
Potato baked				
Ontario, white, baked in skin (Canada)	60	150 g	30	18
Potato, baked, Russet Burbank				
Russet, baked without fat (Canada)	56			
Russet, baked without fat, 45–60 min (USA)	78			
Russet, baked without fat (USA)	94			
Russet, baked without fat (USA)	111			
Average of four studies	85	150 g	30	26
Potato boiled				
Desiree (Australia)	101	150 g	17	17
Nardine (New Zealand)	70	150 g	25	18
Ontario (Canada)	58	150 g	27	16
Pontiac (Australia)	88	150 g	18	16
Prince Edward Island (Canada)	63	150 g	18	11
Sebago (Australia)	87	150 g	17	14
White (Romania)	41	150 g	30	12
White (Canada)	54	150 g	27	15
Type NS (India)	76	150 g	34	26
Type NS refrigerated, reheated (India)	23	150 g	34	8
Potato canned				
Prince Edward Island (Cobi Foods, Canada)	61	150 g	18	11

* Average

FOOD	GI	NOMINAL SERVE SIZE	AVAILABLE CARB PER SERVE	GL PER SERVE
New (Mint Tiny Taters Edgell's, Australia)	65	150 g	18	12
Average of two studies	63	150 g	18	11
Potato, French fries				
French fries, frozen and reheated (Cavendish Farms, Canada)	75	150 g	29	22
Potato instant mashed				
Instant (France)	74			
Instant (Canada)	84*			
Instant (Edgell's, Australia)	86			
Instant (Carnation, Canada)	86			
Instant (USA)	97			
Average of six studies	85	150 g	20	17
Potato, mashed				
Type NS (Canada)	67			
Type NS (South Africa)	71			
Type NS (France)	83			
Prince Edward Island, (Canada)	73	150 g	18	13
Pontiac (Australia)	91	150 g	20	18
Average of five studies	92	150 g	20	18
Potato microwaved				
Pontiac, peeled and microwaved on high for 6–7.5 min (Australia)	79	150 g	18	14
Type NS, microwaved (USA)	82	150 g	33	27
Potato new				
New (Canada)	47			
New (Canada)	54			
New (Canada)	70			
New (Australia)	78			
Average of four studies	62	150 g	21	13

* Average

FOOD	GI	NOMINAL SERVE SIZE	AVAILABLE CARB PER SERVE	GL PER SERVE
Potato steamed				
Potato, peeled, steamed (India)	65	150 g	27	18
Potato dumplings (Italy)	52	150 g	45	24
Potato sweet				
Sweet potato, *Ipomoea batatas* (Australia)	44	150 g	25	11
Sweet potato, (Canada)	48	150 g	34	16
Sweet potato (Canada)	59	150 g	30	18
Sweet potato, kumara (New Zealand)	78	150 g	25	20
Average of five studies	61	150 g	28	17
Pumpkin				
Pumpkin (South Africa)	75	80 g	4	3
Squash				
Squash	[0]	80 g	0	0
Swede				
Swede (rutabaga) (Canada)	72	150 g	10	7
Tapioca				
Tapioca boiled with milk (General Mills, Canada)	81	250 g	18	14
Tapioca (*Manihot utilissima*), steamed one hour (India)	70	250 g	18	12
Taro				
Taro (*Colocasia esculenta*), boiled (Australia)	54			
Taro, boiled (New Zealand)	56			
Average of two studies	55	150 g	8	4
Yam				
Yam, peeled, boiled (New Zealand)	25			
Yam, peeled, boiled (New Zealand)	35			
Yam (Canada)	51			
Average of three studies	37	150 g	36	13

* Average

LOW TO HIGH
GI VALUES

For those people who wish to choose the lowest GI diet possible we've created the following listing in order of GI, ie from lowest to highest. It is also divided into food categories, so that when you want to find a low GI vegetable or a low GI fruit, for example, the information is at your fingertips. This listing may also provide you with new food ideas to try, rather than just checking the GI value of the food you eat.

We have still included some medium and high GI foods as well. As we discuss in *The New Glucose Revolution* you don't need to eat all your carbohydrate from low GI sources. If half of your carbohydrate is from low GI sources you are doing well. If you eat a low GI food at each meal, then your overall GI will be reduced.

Don't forget either that the glycemic load is also included in these lists. In this way you can choose foods with either a low GI and/or a low GL. But don't make the mistake of using GL alone. If you do, you might find yourself eating a diet with very little carbohydrate but a lot of fat, especially saturated fat, and excessive amounts of protein.

FOOD	GI	NOMINAL SERVE SIZE	AVAILABLE CARB PER SERVE	GL PER SERVE
Biscuits				
Snack Right™ Fruit Slice	48	25 g	19	9
Highland Oatmeal™	55	25 g	18	10
Digestives	59*	25 g	16	10
Shredded Wheatmeal™	62	25 g	18	11
Shortbread	64	25 g	16	10
Milk Arrowroot™	69	25 g	18	12
Morning Coffee™	79	25 g	19	15
Bread				
Bürgen® Soy-Lin	36	30 g	9	3
Performax™ (Country Life)	38	30 g	13	5
9-Grain Multi-Grain (Tip Top)	43	30 g	14	11
Bürgen™ Fruit loaf	44	30 g	13	6
Continental fruit loaf	47	30 g	15	7
Ploughman's™ Wholegrain	47	30 g	14	7
Bürgen® Oat Bran & Honey bread	49	40 g	13	7
Bürgen™ Dark/Swiss rye	65	30 g	10	9
Sourdough rye	53	30 g	12	6
Fruit and Spice Loaf (Buttercup)	54	30 g	15	8
Multigrain Spelt wheat Loaf	54	30 g	15	8
Sourdough wheat	54	30 g	14	8
Spelt multigrain bread	54	30 g	12	7
Vogel's Honey & Oats	55	30 g	14	7
Pita bread	57	30 g	17	10
Sunflower and barley bread (Riga)	57	30 g	11	6
Wholemeal rye bread	58*	30 g	14	8
Roggenbrot, (Vogel's)	59	30 g	14	8
Hamburger bun, white	61	30 g	15	9

* Average

FOOD	GI	NOMINAL SERVE SIZE	AVAILABLE CARB PER SERVE	GL PER SERVE
Rice bread, high-amylose Doongara rice	61	30 g	12	7
Pain au lait	63	60 g	32	20
Ploughman's™ wholemeal	64	30 g	13	9
Barley flour bread	67	30 g	13	9
Helga's™ Classic Seed Loaf	68	30 g	14	9
Helga's™ traditional wholemeal bread	70	30 g	13	9
Melba toast	70	30 g	23	16
White bread	70	30 g	14	10
Bagel, white	72	70 g	35	25
Rice bread, low-amylose Calrose rice	72	30 g	12	8
Kaiser rolls	73	30 g	16	12
Lebanese bread, white	75	30 g	16	12
Blackbread (Riga)	76	30 g	13	10
Wholemeal bread	77	30 g	12	9
Gluten-free multigrain bread	79	30 g	13	10
Wonderwhite™ (Buttercup)	80	30 g	14	11
Schinkenbrot (Riga)	86	30 g	14	12
Baguette, white	95	30 g	15	14
Breakfast bars				
Fruity-Bix™ bar, wild berry	51	30 g	19	9
Fruity-Bix™ bar, fruit and nut	56	30 g	19	10
Sustain™ bar	57	30 g	25	14
Rice Bubble Treat™ bar	63	30 g	24	15
Crunchy Nut Cornflakes™ bar	72	30 g	26	19
K-Time Just Right™ bar	72	30 g	24	17
K-Time Strawberry Crunch™ bar	77	30 g	25	19
Fibre Plus™ bar	78	30 g	23	18

* Average

FOOD	GI	NOMINAL SERVE SIZE	AVAILABLE CARB PER SERVE	GL PER SERVE
Breakfast cereal				
Rice Bran, extruded	19	30 g	14	3
All-Bran™	30	30 g	15	5
All-Bran Soy 'n' Fibre™	33	30 g	14	4
Guardian™	37	30 g	12	5
All-Bran Fruit 'n' Oats™	39	30 g	17	7
Muesli, gluten-free	39	30 g	19	7
Ultra-bran™, soy and linseed	41	30 g	13	5
Muesli, toasted (Purina)	43	30 g	17	7
Healthwise™ for heart health	48	30 g	19	9
Komplete™	48	30 g	21	10
Muesli, Natural	48*	30 g	18	8
Soytana™ (Vogel's)	49	45 g	25	12
Traditional porridge oats	51	250 g	21	11
Special K™	54	30 g	21	11
Frosties™	55	30 g	26	15
Porridge, made from whole rolled oats	55*	250 g	21	11
Hi-Bran Weet-Bix™ with soy and linseed	57	30 g	16	9
Oat bran Weet-Bix™	57	30 g	20	11
Mini Wheats™, whole wheat	58	30 g	21	12
Just Right™	60	30 g	22	13
Soy Tasty™	60	30 g	20	12
Hi-Bran Weet-Bix™	61	30 g	17	10
Just Right Just Grains™	62	30 g	23	14
Sultana Goldies™	65	30 g	21	13
Healthwise™ for bowel health	66	30 g	18	12
Instant porridge	66	250 g	26	17
Nutrigrain™	66*	30 g	15	10

* Average

FOOD	GI	NOMINAL SERVE SIZE	AVAILABLE CARB PER SERVE	GL PER SERVE
Good Start™, muesli wheat biscuits	68	30 g	20	14
Vita-Brits™	68	30 g	20	13
Sustain™	68	30 g	22	15
Froot Loops™	69	30 g	26	18
Weet-Bix™	69	30 g	17	12
Lite-Bix™, no added sugar	70	30 g	20	14
Pop Tarts™, chocolate	70	50 g	36	25
Whole wheat Goldies™	70	30 g	20	14
Golden Wheats™	71	30 g	23	16
Honey Smacks™	71	30 g	23	16
Cornflakes, Crunchy Nut™	72	30 g	24	17
Honey Goldies™	72	30 g	21	15
Mini Wheats™, blackcurrant	72	30 g	21	15
Wheat-bites™	72	30 g	25	18
Sultana Bran™	73	30 g	19	14
Bran Flakes™	74	30 g	18	13
Shredded Wheat	75	30 g	20	15
Coco Pops™	77	30 g	26	20
Cornflakes™	77	30 g	25	20
Honey Rice Bubbles™	77	30 g	27	20
Oat 'n' Honey Bake™	77	30 g	17	13
Corn Pops™	80	30 g	26	21
Puffed Wheat	80	30 g	21	17
Rice Bubbles™	87	30 g	26	22
Cereal grains				
Pearl Barley, boiled	25	150 g	32	8
Rye, whole kernels	34	50 g	38	13
Wheat, whole kernels, cooked	41	50 g	34	14
Cracked wheat (bulghur), cooked	48*	150 g	26	12
Sweet corn	48	150 g	30	14

* Average

FOOD	GI	NOMINAL SERVE SIZE	AVAILABLE CARB PER SERVE	GL PER SERVE
Koshikari (Japanese) white rice, boiled	48	150 g	42	20
Parboiled, Doongara rice, boiled	50	150 g	39	19
Buckwheat, boiled	54	150 g	30	16
Wheat, quick-cooking kernels	54	150 g	47	25
Rice, brown, boiled	55	150 g	33	18
Semolina, cooked	55	150 g	11	6
Doongara rice, white	56	150 g	39	22
Long grain rice, boiled	56	150 g	41	23
Basmati rice, boiled (Mahatma, Australia)	58	150 g	38	22
Couscous	65	150 g	33	21
Barley, rolled	66	50 g	38	25
Doongara rice, brown, boiled	66	150 g	37	24
Arborio, risotto rice, boiled	69	150 g	53	36
Cornmeal, boiled	69	150 g	13	9
Pelde brown rice, boiled	76	150 g	38	29
Sunbrown rice Quick™, boiled	80	150 g	38	31
Calrose rice, white, medium grain, boiled	83	150 g	43	36
Calrose rice, brown, boiled	87	150 g	38	33
Instant rice, white, cooked 6 min	87	150 g	42	36
Parboiled rice, Sungold	87	150 g	39	34
Sungold rice, Pelde, parboiled	87	150 g	43	37
Pelde, white	93	150 g	43	40
Instant Doongara rice, white	94	150 g	42	35
Jasmine rice	109	150 g	42	46
Crackers				
Jatz™	55	25 g	17	10
Vita-wheat™, original, crispbread	55	25 g	19	10
Rye crispbread	64*	25 g	16	11

* Average

FOOD	GI	NOMINAL SERVE SIZE	AVAILABLE CARB PER SERVE	GL PER SERVE
Breton wheat crackers	67	25 g	14	10
Sao™, plain square crackers	70	25 g	17	12
Kavli™ Norwegian Crispbread	71	25 g	16	12
Water cracker	78	25 g	18	14
Puffed Crispbread	81	25 g	19	15
Puffed rice cakes	82	25 g	21	17
Dairy products				
Yoghurt, low fat, fruit, aspartame, Ski™	14	200 g	13	2
Milk, low fat, chocolate, no added sugar	24	250 ml	15	3
Milk, full-fat, fresh	31	250 ml	12	4
Yoghurt, low fat, fruit, sugar, Ski™	33	200 g	31	10
Mousse, reduced fat, from mix	34*	50 g	10	4
Ice-cream, Prestige Light™, traditional toffee (Norco, Australia)	37	50 g	14	5
Ice-cream, Ultra chocolate, 15% fat (Sara Lee, Australia)	37	50 g	9	4
Ice-cream, Prestige™, golden macadamia (Norco, Australia)	37	50 g	9	3
Custard	38*	100 g	16	6
Ice-cream, French vanilla, 16% fat (Sara Lee, Australia)	38	50 g	9	3
Reduced-fat yoghurt drink, Vaalia™, passionfruit	38	200 g	29	11
Yoghurt, no-fat, Strawberry, Vaalia, with sugar	38	150 ml	22	8
Yoghurt, no-fat, Wildberry, Vaalia, with sugar	38	150 ml	22	8

* Average

FOOD	GI	NOMINAL SERVE SIZE	AVAILABLE CARB PER SERVE	GL PER SERVE
Yoghurt, no-fat, Mango, Vaalia, with sugar	39	150 ml	25	10
Yoghurt, no-fat, French Vanilla, Vaalia, with sugar	40	150 ml	27	10
Milk, chocolate, sugar-sweetened	43	50 ml	28	12
Ice-cream, vanilla, Peter's Light and Creamy	44	150 ml	13	6
Ice-cream, vanilla, Prestige Light™ (Norco, Australia)	47	50 g	10	5
Ice-cream, vanilla	50	50 g	6	3
Ice-cream, regular	61	50 g	13	8
Fruit				
Cherries	22	120 g	12	3
Grapefruit	25	120 g	11	3
Pear halves, canned in reduced-sugar syrup (SPC Lite)	25	120 g	14	4
Apple, dried	29	60 g	34	10
Prunes, pitted	29	60 g	33	10
Apricots, dried	31*	60 g	27	8
Peach, canned in natural juice	38	120 g	11	4
Apple	38*	120 g	15	6
Pears	38	120 g	11	4
Plum	3*	120 g	12	5
Strawberries	40	120 g	3	1
Oranges	42	120 g	11	5
Peach	42*	120 g	8	5
Pear halves, canned in natural juice	43	120 g	13	5
Grapes	46*	120 g	18	8
Mango	51*	120 g	15	8
Banana	52*	120 g	26	13

* Average

FOOD	GI	NOMINAL SERVE SIZE	AVAILABLE CARB PER SERVE	GL PER SERVE
Kiwi fruit	53*	120 g	12	6
Sultanas	56	60 g	45	25
Grapes, black	59	120 g	18	11
Paw paw	56	120 g	8	5
Pineapple	59*	120 g	13	7
Figs	61	60 g	26	16
Raisins	64	60 g	44	28
Rockmelon	65	120 g	6	4
Watermelon	72	120 g	6	4
Lychee, canned in syrup, drained	79	120 g	20	16
Dates, dried	103	60 g	40	42
Fruit juice				
Apple juice, pure, cloudy (Wild About Fruit, Australia)	37	250 ml	28	10
Tomato juice, canned	38	250 ml	9	4
Apple juice, unsweetened	40	250 ml	29	12
Carrot juice	43	250 ml	23	10
Apple juice, pure, clear (Wild About Fruit, Australia)	44	250 ml	30	13
Pineapple juice, unsweetened	46	250 ml	34	16
Grapefruit juice, unsweetened	48	250 ml	22	11
Cranberry juice cocktail	52	250 ml	31	16
Orange juice, unsweetened	50	250 ml	19	9
Legumes				
Soy beans, dried, boiled	18*	150 g	6	1
Peas, dried, boiled	22	150 g	9	2
Lentils, red, dried, boiled	26*	150 g	18	5
Chickpeas, dried, boiled	28*	150 g	24	7
Kidney beans, dried, cooked	28*	150 g	25	7
Lentils, boiled	29	150 g	18	5
Lentils, green, dried, boiled	30*	150 g	17	5

* Average

FOOD	GI	NOMINAL SERVE SIZE	AVAILABLE CARB PER SERVE	GL PER SERVE
Butter Beans, boiled	31*	150 g	20	6
Mung bean, dried, boiled	42	150 g	17	7
Lima beans, baby, cooked	32	150 g	30	10
Split peas, yellow, boiled	32	150 g	19	6
Haricot/navy beans, pressure cooked	38	150 g	31	12
Marrowfat peas	39	150 g	19	7
Blackeyed beans, boiled	42*	150 g	21	12
Baked Beans, canned	48*	150 g	15	7
Meat				
Beef	[0]	120 g	0	0
Lamb	[0]	120 g	0	0
Pork	[0]	120 g	0	0
Salami	[0]	120 g	0	0
Tuna	[0]	120 g	0	0
Veal	[0]	120 g	0	0
Pasta and noodles				
Spaghetti, wholemeal, boiled	37*	180 g	42	16
Mung bean noodles	39	180 g	45	18
Ravioli	39	180 g	38	15
Fettucine, egg, boiled	40	180 g	46	18
Rice noodles	40	180 g	39	15
Spaghetti, white, boiled	42*	180 g	47	20
Spirali, durum wheat, white, boiled	43	180 g	44	19
Spaghetti, white, boiled 10–15 min	44*	180 g	48	21
Instant noodles	47	180 g	40	19
Macaroni	47	180 g	48	23
Linguine	49*	180 g	47	23

* Average

FOOD	GI	NOMINAL SERVE SIZE	AVAILABLE CARB PER SERVE	GL PER SERVE
Spaghetti, white, boiled 20 min	61*	180 g	44	27
Udon noodles, plain	62	180 g	48	30
Macaroni and Cheese, boxed (Kraft, Canada)	64	180 g	51	32
Gnocchi	68	180 g	48	33
Spaghetti, gluten-free, canned in tomato sauce	68	220 g	27	19
Rice pasta, brown, boiled	92	180 g	38	35
Potato				
Yam	37	150 g	36	13
Sweet potato	44	150 g	25	11
Taro	55	150 g	8	4
Boiled potatoes, Ontario	58	150 g	27	16
Baked potato, Ontario	60	150 g	30	18
New potato	62	150 g	21	13
Canned potato, new	65	150 g	18	12
Potato, peeled, steamed	65	150 g	27	18
Swede	72	150 g	10	7
French fries	75	150 g	29	22
Pontiac, peeled and microwaved on high for 6–7.5 min	79	150 g	18	14
Baked, Russet Burbank potato	85	150 g	30	26
Instant mashed potato	85	150 g	20	17
Boiled potatoes, Sebago	87	150 g	17	14
Boiled potatoes, Pontiac	88	150 g	18	16
Mashed potato, Pontiac	91	150 g	20	18
Boiled potatoes, Desiree	101	150 g	17	17
Rice				
Parboiled rice, Doongara	50	150 g	39	19
Rice, brown	55	150 g	33	18
Doongara rice, white	56	150 g	39	22

* Average

FOOD	GI	NOMINAL SERVE SIZE	AVAILABLE CARB PER SERVE	GL PER SERVE
Long grain rice, boiled	56	150 g	41	23
Basmati rice, boiled	58	150 g	42	24
Doongara rice, brown	66	150 g	37	24
Arborio, risotto rice, boiled	69	150 g	43	29
Pelde rice, brown	76	150 g	38	29
Sunbrown Quick™ rice	80	150 g	38	31
Calrose rice, white, medium grain, boiled	83	150 g	42	35
Calrose rice brown	87	150 g	40	35
Instant rice, white	87	150 g	42	36
Parboiled rice, Sungold	87	150 g	39	34
Sungold rice, Pelde, parboiled	87	150 g	43	37
Pelde rice, white	93	150 g	43	40
Instant Doongara rice, white	94	150 g	42	35
Jasmine rice, long grain	109	150 g	42	46
Snacks				
M & M's®, peanut	33	30 g	17	6
Nutella®	33	20 g	12	4
Fruity Bitz	39*	15 g	12	4
Snickers Bar®	41	60 g	36	15
Corn chips, plain, salted	42	50 g	25	11
Chocolate, milk, plain	43*	50 g	28	12
Chocolate, white, Milky Bar®	44	50 g	29	13
Twix bar®	44	60 g	39	17
Apricot filled fruit bar	50	50 g	34	17
Potato crisps, plain, salted	57	50 g	18	10
Heinz Kidz™ Fruit Fingers	61	30 g	20	12
Muesli bar, with dried fruit	61	30 g	21	13
Mars Bar®	62	60 g	40	25
Life Savers®	70	30 g	30	21
Pop Tarts™, chocolate	70	50 g	35	24

* Average

FOOD	GI	NOMINAL SERVE SIZE	AVAILABLE CARB PER SERVE	GL PER SERVE
Skittles®	70	50 g	45	32
Popcorn, cooked in microwave	72	20 g	11	8
Twisties™	74	50 g	29	22
Jelly beans	78	30 g	28	22
Pretzels, oven baked	83	30 g	20	16
Burger Rings™	90	50 g	31	28
Real Fruit Bars™, strawberry	90	30 g	26	23
Roll-Ups®	99	30 g	25	24
Soft drinks				
Coca Cola®, soft drink	53	250 ml	26	14
Solo™, lemon squash, soft drink	58	250 ml	29	17
Cordial, orange	66	250 ml	20	13
Fanta®, orange soft drink	68	250 ml	34	23
Lucozade®, original	95	250 ml	42	40
Soups				
Tomato soup	38	250 ml	17	6
Minestrone, Country Ladle™	39	250 ml	18	7
Lentil, canned	44	250 ml	21	9
Split Pea	60	250 ml	27	16
Black Bean	64	250 ml	27	17
Green Pea, canned	66	250 ml	41	27
Sports drinks				
Sustagen Sport®	43	250 ml	49	21
Isostar®	70	250 ml	18	13
Sports Plus®	74	250 ml	17	13
Gatorade®	78	250 ml	15	12
Sugars				
Fructose	19	10 g	10	2
Yellow box honey	35	25 g	18	6
Stringy Bark honey	44	25 g	21	9
Lactose	46	10 g	10	5

* Average

FOOD	GI	NOMINAL SERVE SIZE	AVAILABLE CARB PER SERVE	GL PER SERVE
Red Gum honey	46	25 g	18	8
Iron Bark honey	48	25 g	15	7
Yapunya honey	52	25 g	17	9
Pure Capilano™ honey	58	25 g	21	12
Sucrose	68*	10 g	10	6
Commercial Blend honey	62	25 g	18	11
Salvation Jane honey	64	25 g	15	10
Commercial Blend honey	72	25 g	13	9
Glucose	100	10 g	10	10
Maltose	105	10 g	10	11
Vegetables				
Carrots, peeled, boiled	41*	80 g	5	2
Green peas, boiled	48	80 g	7	3
Corn on the cob, sweet, boiled	48*	80 g	16	8
Beetroot, canned	64	80 g	7	5
Broad beans, cooked	79	80 g	11	9
Parsnips	97	80 g	12	12
Artichokes	[0]	80 g	0	0
Avocado	[0]	80 g	0	0
Bokchoy	[0]	80 g	0	0
Broccoli	[0]	80 g	0	0
Cabbage	[0]	80 g	0	0
Capsicum	[0]	80 g	0	0
Cauliflower	[0]	80 g	0	0
Celery	[0]	80 g	0	0
Cucumber	[0]	80 g	0	0
French beans (runner beans)	[0]	80 g	0	0
Leafy vegetables (spinach, rocket etc)	[0]	80 g	0	0
Lettuce	[0]	80 g	0	0

* Average

About the authors

Professor Jennie Brand-Miller is Professor of Human Nutrition in the Human Nutrition Unit, School of Molecular and Microbial Biosciences at the University of Sydney, and President of the Nutrition Society of Australia. She has taught postgraduate students of nutrition and dietetics at the University of Sydney for over 24 years and currently leads a team of 12 research scientists. Professor Brand-Miller was recently awarded a Clunies Ross National Science and Technology Medal for her work in championing a new approach to nutrition and the management of blood glucose.

Kaye Foster-Powell, is an accredited practising dietitian with extensive experience in diabetes management. A graduate of the University of Sydney (BSc, Master of Nutrition and Dietitics), she has conducted research into the glycemic index of foods and its practical applications over the last 15 years. Currently she is a dietitian with Wentworth Area Diabetes Services and provides consultancy on all aspects of the glycemic index. Her most recent book is the bestselling *The GI Factor*, recently updated and republished as *The New Glucose Revolution*.

Dr Susanna Holt works closely with Professor Jennie Brand-Miller as the Research Manager of Sydney University's Glycemic Index Research Service (SUGiRS). Susanna is also a qualified dietitian and nutrition consultant.

A Guide for Trainees in General Practice

Second Edition

John Fry CBE, MD, FRCS, FRCGP
General Practitioner, Kent

Eric Gambrill FRCGP
General Practitioner, Associate Regional Adviser, Sussex

Martin Godfrey MB, CHB, MRCGP
Editor, General Practitioner Magazine

Peter Martin FRCGP
General Practitioner, Essex

Alistair Moulds FRCGP
General Practitioner, Associate Regional Adviser, Essex

Gillian Strube MB, BS, DCHS
General Practitioner, Sussex

Heinemann Medical Books

Heinemann Medical Books

An imprint of Heinemann Professional Publishing Ltd
Halley Court, Jordan Hill, Oxford OX2 8EJ
OXFORD LONDON SINGAPORE NAIROBI
IBADAN KINGSTON

First published 1982
Reprinted 1983, 1986

Second edition 1989

British Library Cataloguing in Publication Data

Guide for trainees in general practice
  2nd ed.
  1. General practice
  I. Fry, John, *1922*-
  362.1′72

ISBN 0-433-10919-X

Typeset by Lasertext Ltd, Manchester and Printed by
Thomson Litho Ltd, East Kilbride, Scotland

Preface

This second edition has been completely re-written because of the changes that have, and are taking place, in general practice in the National Health Service.

General practice is the most popular first choice of young medical graduates and over one-half of all doctors go into general practice.

General practice is a 'specialty', a special field of medical practice now requiring a mandatory three year period of training.

General practice has very many differences from hospital practice and it is a major transition for the young doctor requiring a fresh re–orientation on doctor-patient relations, the morbidity spectrum and management of situations unmet in hospitals, and also the need for organization and administration of a practice.

Our Guide aims to help in this transition in the process of training and preparation for independent practice as a principal.

We cover the field of describing the nature of general practice, its organization, relations with other colleagues, the law, ethics and behaviour, and an understanding of common bread-and-butter conditions, as well as care for chronic illness.

We are grateful that our first edition was successful enough to require two reprintings, and we hope that this new re-written second edition will help generations of GPs to prepare to enjoy their lifework in practice.

John Fry

Part One
What is General Practice?

Chapter 1

Special features of general practice

General practice, or primary care, is an essential and inevitable part of medical care in all countries. Sandwiched between the self-care provided for themselves by individuals and families and the specialist services in local hospitals, general practice serves as the first point of medical contact for the public, except for some accidents and emergencies and for those with sexually transmitted diseases who may go direct to the relevant hospital departments.

There are some distinct differences from hospital practice.

DIRECT ACCESS

Patients may consult their family doctor (general practitioner, GP) when they think it necessary. Hospital specialists can be seen only through referral by a family doctor.

LOCAL AVAILABILITY

General practice premises have to be reasonably accessible to patients, ideally within pram-push walking distance, although at least two-thirds of all households now have access to a private car.

PRESENTATION OF ILLNESS

Whereas patients' problems have been pre-packaged by the GP into surgical, medical, psychiatric, obstetric, gynaecological, etc., before referral to hospital specialists, in general practice itself the doctor is presented with vague collections of symptoms. These have to be assessed and diagnosed as some meaningful clinical condition before being managed. First contact care demands knowledge, skill, sympathetic understanding and experience.

SMALL COMMUNITY

The population base (practice list) of one GP is about 2000 patients of whom only 5 to 10 per cent move in any one year. A district general hospital serves a population of about 250,000.

CONTINUING CARE

In the fairly small and static population, patients and doctors can get to know each other well. A practitioner who starts in his practice at 30 years of age will work in it for up to 40 years. Such long-term continuing care is the hallmark of British general practice. This is in contrast to the transient and episodic nature of the care given in hospitals.

THE NATURE AND INCIDENCE OF DISEASE

A GP with 2000 patients can expect to meet and treat only those diseases that occur in a population of this size. A district general hospital covering a population of 200,000 plus will see 100 times as many of hospital-type conditions. Thus, the GP will see three to five acute abdomens a year while local surgical units will see 300 to 500. Two-thirds of disease in general practice is minor, one-quarter is chronic, and one-twentieth major. In hospitals the proportions are reversed.

OPPORTUNITIES

Under the National Health Service (NHS) patients are 'registered' with their GP. It is therefore possible to construct an age–sex register for the population at risk and to carry out short-term and long-term audits and research studies into the course and outcome of common diseases.

Chapter 2

The work of the practice

The bulk of the work of the practice is carried out in consultations at the surgery and on home visits. The GP also spends time in the practice's children's clinic and on immunizations, antenatal and postnatal care, family planning and cervical cytology, medical check-ups, insurance examinations, repeat prescribing, writing referral letters and reports, administration, work outside the practice, and teaching and learning.

CONSULTATIONS

Over 80 per cent of face-to-face patient contacts occur in consultations in the practice premises.

Purposes of the consultation

- To provide an opportunity for the patient to seek the doctor's advice and help for new problems and for the continuing care of chronic problems through follow-up attendances.
- To allow the patient to ventilate feelings and emotions about himself/herself or others.
- To use the patient's visit to promote personal health education on lifestyle and to promote uptake of preventative procedures.
- To chat generally about the patient's family.

Some objectives for the doctor in the consultation:
- To establish a good rapport.
- To find the reason for the consultation (this may not be easy!).
- To determine who is the patient.
- To obtain any necessary information by oral and physical examination.
- To allow the patient to express feelings, complaints and ideas about the nature of the problem.
- To share information with the patient.

- To agree a management plan with the patient.
- To implement the plan.
- To use some time for education, prevention and screening.
- To be economic and realistic in the use of time.
- To terminate the consultation kindly and efficiently.

All these objectives may not be achievable in one contact but may well be so over a series of contacts, which is the norm in practice.

The GP consultation differs from a hospital consultation in that:

- The patient has free access to the doctor.
- The patient can bring any problem he/she wishes.
- The problems are often ill-defined.
- The doctor is obliged to provide any necessary treatment.
- The consultation may develop over a series of contacts so it is not necessary to get through all the business at the first meeting. Time can be used as a tool.
- What ever the outcome of the consultation, the GP has to have a continuing relationship with and a responsibility for that patient.

Conducting the consultation

The *history* is the most important part of the consultation. General practice involves a long-term follow-up of the same patients over many years. The personal, family and past histories evolve and become well known to the GP. The formal type of history-taking has to be modified to suit the shorter consultations of general practice. However, the GP must always allow the patient the time and opportunity to express fears and feelings.

The *examination* has to be selective but never skimped. At least once every few years records should be made of height, weight, blood pressure, peak flow rates and urinalysis.

The *action* must include clear and simple explanation to the patient of your diagnosis based on any pathology. Use the opportunity to advise the patient on a healthy lifestyle and give instructions on what can be done by the patient to help himself. Investigations should only be organized when considered relevant and necessary.

The *treatment*, whether it is a prescription or advice, should be given with clear instructions on what it is hoped to achieve, how to take it, actions and possible side effects, and expected course and outcome of the condition. Do not forget to say when and if you want to see the patient again or whether you want the patient to telephone through a progress report.

Whatever the problem is and whatever the management, sure ways to success in general practice are to be caring, sympathetic, interested, unhurried and as optimistic and cheerful as possible.

Appointment systems

A good appointment system has to benefit patients, doctors and receptionists by organizing the distribution of the work and shortening waiting times. It cannot be used to limit patient demand. It has to be flexible to meet unexpected urgent situations.

Appointment systems are particularly useful for increasing patient compliance and for follow-up checks on diabetes, hypertension, immunization, antenatal care, etc.

A good appointment system should:

- Provide enough appointments to avoid patients having to wait more than one or two days to see a doctor of their choice.
- Be flexible so as to cope with variations in workload throughout the year.
- Allow for emergencies (as perceived by the patient).
- Make patients feel welcome.

HOME VISITS

Home visiting is still an important part of British general practice. It is much less frequent than in the past because there is less serious acute disease managed at home, better transport for children and adults to be brought to the surgery, better medical treatment (such as antibiotics, drugs for cardiac and respiratory conditions that keep patients ambulant), and patient expectation of a visit is less. There is also the delegation of chronic sick visiting by GPs to nurses.

The advantages of home visits

- The doctor is given the privilege of entering the patient's home and observing social standards and conditions.
- The problems of the handicapped and elderly can be assessed.
- They promote better doctor–patient relationships.

The disadvantages of home visits

- Home visits take three to four times as much time as surgery consultations (most by in travel time).
- The lack of facilities for diagnosis and treatment.

Reluctance or refusal to do a home visit is the most frequent reason for complaint about a GP to the Family Practitioner Committees (FPCs) and may even lead to a hearing at the General Medical Council. Therefore, when in doubt *visit* rather than refuse.

THE TELEPHONE

The telephone is a double-edged tool. It is the usual method of communication for emergencies and is increasingly used to obtain advice and information and to order repeat prescriptions. As four out of five households now have telephones, the number of calls to the practice increases.

Advantages of using the telephone

- To give advice on minor problems.
- To take messages for prescriptions and avoid congestion in the practice premises.
- To give results of tests and other information.

Good telephone techniques

- A kind, gentle, considerate manner helps for a smooth interaction.
- A well-meaning tone makes advice more likely to be accepted.
- Anxious patients are likely to be aggressive on the telephone. Do not react likewise. Patiently try to sort out the problem rather than remonstrate.
- Avoid direct refusals to requests for home visits, discuss the situation but leave the final decision to the caller. Visit first, then educate later as necessary.

REPEAT PRESCRIBING AND PRESCRIBING FOR THE UNSEEN PATIENT

About a half of all prescriptions (items) are written for 'unseen patients'. Most of the prescriptions are repeats but some are in response to a telephone request for help.

Warnings

- Be careful when prescribing for an unseen patient. If for a minor illness, is a prescription really necessary? If the condition is bad enough for a specific drug, e.g. an antibiotic, then should not the patient be seen?
- Always record all prescriptions given.
- Personal prescription cards make repeat prescribing easier.
- Ensure that patients on long-term therapy are reviewed at regular intervals.

OUT OF HOURS COVER

The NHS contract specifies 24-hour responsibility but this is a practical impossibility. However, whatever arrangements are made, the patients' GP is responsible for ensuring that there is alternative medical cover when he is not available.

Possible systems

- Single-handed practitioners or small groups may make reciprocal arrangements with neighbouring practices.
- Larger groups may organize in-practice rotas.
- Commercial deputizing services employ doctors to provide cover and charge appropriate fees.
- In a few areas local doctors organize their own deputizing services on a cooperative basis.

FPCs are now empowered to supervise the work of local deputizing services and to check that individual GPs do not overuse them.

WORK OUTSIDE THE PRACTICE

About three out of four GPs have regular paid employment outside their NHS general practices.

Variety of work

- Hospital appointments as clinical assistants or hospital practitioners.
- Private practices.

- Medical officers to schools, homes, clubs, voluntary organizations and industry.
- Medical examinations for insurance, government agencies, companies, sports groups.
- Teaching trainees, undergraduates, nurses or lay groups.
- Writing.

Chapter 3

Types of practice

General practice allows individual practitioners a wide choice of where to practice, with whom and how.

SINGLE-HANDED PRACTICE

Single-handed practice was usual before the NHS, now only one out of every ten GPs work in this way. Its advantages are that one is truly one's own boss and patients have complete one-to-one care. The disadvantages are arranging out-of-hours cover and holidays.

GROUP PRACTICE

Group practice is currently most popular with a continuing trend towards larger partnerships. One-third of all GPs now work in groups of five or more. Advantages are sharing of work, resources and expenses and scope for more of the newer methods and techniques such as screening, special clinics, minor surgery and larger practice teams. Disadvantages are problems of communication within the practice and difficulties may be faced by patients in larger organizations.

HEALTH CENTRES

There are now 1200 health centres built by local authorities who rent them out to GPs. Advantages are that premises are provided and maintained and rent is met through the NHS. Disadvantages are limited freedom.

GENERAL PRACTITIONERS' LISTS

There are now over 30,000 GP principals for the UK population of 56.5 million, i.e., one GP to 1550 people. Correspondingly, there are 18,000 NHS consultants.

Because of inflation of practice lists the average number of patients registered per GP is 1950. List sizes per GP in Scotland (1644) have always been less than in England (2032). Regionally in England, the highest list size is in South West Thames (2185) and lowest in South West England (1905).

The number of GPs is increasing by about 500 each year, and the average list size is falling by 50 patients per GP each year. At present, 20 per cent of GPs are women, but the proportion is expected to be almost 50 per cent by the year 2000.

Part Two
Preparing for Training

Chapter 4

Why choose general practice?

This is not an easy question to answer since everyone has a whole host of reasons why they choose general practice. Some are public while others are very private.

THE GP AS A PRACTITIONER OF MEDICINE

GPs can practise pretty well the whole gamut of medicine should they so wish. No other specialty has such a wide remit in seeing and treating everything from pregnant women and young children to the mentally ill, the very old and the plain unwell. Should you have doubts about leaving behind parts of your medical training then general practice will allow you to remain something of a jack of all trades.

General practice medicine is very different from that seen in hospital practice. General practice medicine is carried out at a much lower key, it is less immediate, more considered and, some might say, less demanding. Most of the patients seen will have chronic, subacute, maybe downright trivial illnesses and you may see several a day for whom you are unable to give a diagnosis. Dealing with these types of problems requires special skills, and in developing these skills the GP gains his/her own unique rewards.

General practice more than any other specialty allows the doctor to prevent disease, not just treat it.

THE GP AS A MEMBER OF A COMMUNITY

The GP has the ability to see not only patients, but their families, their friends, maybe even their employers, and to see them in their own environment. This enables the GP to have a unique view of the whole patient – something usually denied to the hospital practitioner.

General practice allows a doctor to really become part of a community rather than look on at a distance (as occurs in hospital medicine). As a GP you may spend the greater part of your life in the community you choose to practise within, thus you rapidly become a respected member of it.

General practice may allow you and your family to live in the area of the country, in the type of environment, you have always wanted. Many young GPs would still like to see themselves in the 'Dr Finlay' mould.

THE GP AS AN INDEPENDENT CONTRACTOR TO THE NHS

As a GP you are a small business man or woman. You will have the responsibilities of an employer (of receptionists and ancillary staff). You will have to deal with accounts. You may even have to build or update your practice premises. For this you are well paid and indeed can control your income to a degree that may be difficult for someone practising wholly within the NHS.

You are your own boss as to when and for how long (within limits) you practice each week. You may eschew the onerous on-call rotas that ruin the lives of so many hospital doctors.

And all this may be gained without so much as looking at another exam; all you need to do is satisfactorily complete a three-year vocational training course and by the age of about 28 you are a principal. Although not very laudable, these are just as much reasons for some to enter general practice, especially those unsure of their abilities, as many of the others mentioned above.

As a woman, it may be easier to be a mother and continue in general practice part-time than it would be in any other specialty.

COMMON COMPLAINTS

As with any other job, the realities do not always match up to the expectations. In order to enter general practice with your eyes open, here are some of the more common complaints held by practising GPs.

The GP as a practitioner of medicine

Many GPs get sick and tired of seeing a stream of trivial conditions, most of which they know will improve whatever they do. Many yearn for the sort of excitement they rightly or wrongly remember as being part of hospital life.

The GP as a member of the community

Thirty years is a very long time to be tied to one area. Although it is possible to move, with increasing competition for jobs some GPs feel they are stuck in a rut. Also, being a pillar of the community can be hard work – some doctors wish they could let their hair down a little more easily.

The GP as an independent contractor to the NHS

Being your own boss can bring with it a new string of problems. All in all, general practice, like any other job is what you make of it. If you approach it with the right attitude, and you are prepared to devote a lot of time and energy to what is going to be your life's work, then the rewards are beyond compare.

Chapter 5

How to train

MANDATORY VOCATIONAL TRAINING

Since 16 August 1982, a three-year full-time vocational training course, completed within a seven-year period, has been mandatory for anyone wishing to enter general practice.

Training must be made up as follows:

- One year spent as a trainee GP with an approved trainer.
- At least one year involved in at least two of the following six-month hospital appointments:
  General medicine
  Geriatrics
  Obstetrics and/or gynaecology
  Paediatrics
  Psychiatry
  Accident and emergency medicine, or general surgery
  The entire hospital experience may, if desired, be confined to just two of the above.
- Up to a year may be spent in one or more of a wide range of other approved hospital or community medicine posts.
- Part-time posts can count towards the overall experience providing this is no less than half-time, and providing that the total of three years is still fulfilled.
- Equivalent experience attained in a number of ways can also be counted. This includes posts held overseas, electives and occupational health work.

After each hospital post has been completed the trainee must get form VTR/2 signed by their consultant and stamped by the hospital. This shows the job has been completed satisfactorily.

After satisfactory completion of the GP year, form VTR/1 must be signed by the trainer and then forwarded to the regional adviser for verification of his/her signature.

All forms must then be bundled together and sent to the Joint Committee for Postgraduate Training in General Practice (JCPTGP),

14 Princes Gate, London SW7 1PU (telephone 01 581 3232).

This is best done just before the completion of your last post (not more than four weeks before). This will enable the JCPTGP to issue a JCPTGP certificate proving that you have in fact completed the prescribed general practice vocational training course. The certificate will be forwarded to the Medical Practices Committee and this will finally allow you to practise as a fully fledged GP.

The JCPTGP certificate need not be used at once and can be retained as proof of training for the future. If a certificate is not issued then an appeal may be made to the JCPTGP.

STRUCTURE AND ORGANIZATION OF VOCATIONAL TRAINING

The Joint Committee on Postgraduate Training in General Practice

The JCPTGP was set up in 1975 by the Royal College of General Practitioners (RCGP) and the General Medical Services Committee of the British Medical Association.

It has 24 members drawn from all areas of medical education and exists to monitor training and training programmes and to advise on the standards required for training. It also processes and issues certificates of prescribed equivalent experience.

The committee conducts regular two-yearly visits to all regions to monitor their training arrangements.

Postgraduate adviser

Vocational training throughout the country is divided up into separate regions and controlled by the General Practice Subcommittees of autonomous Postgraduate Medical Education Committees. The key organizational position in each region is filled by the Regional Postgraduate Adviser who oversees everything that goes on in vocational training.

The adviser may be approached about vacancies in that region's training schemes, as a source of information or as a receiver of complaints. A list of who the advisers are and where they may be contacted is available from the RCGP.

Course organizer

Course organizers are GPs who organize and oversee each individual vocational training scheme (see below). They must be trainers. They are particularly involved in the planning and day-to-day running of the course, liaising with the regional postgraduate adviser and the individual trainers.

GP trainer

Trainers are appointed by the General Practice Subcommittee of the Regional Postgraduate Medical Education Committee. They must have had at least three years experience in general practice, and be judged 'ready, willing and able' to be a trainer by the Committee. They must also work in a practice which is assessed as being suitable for training (assessments of suitability are made at regular intervals).

A trainer is appointed initially for two years and then for three-year periods.

Formal vocational training schemes

These schemes are organized by the Regional Postgraduate Committees and provide a coordinated package of hospital rotations together with a choice of GP training posts.

The advantage of these schemes is that trainees are spared the necessity of applying for new posts every six months and can thus plan their life – where they are going to live, etc. Trainees are also assured that the posts are educationally approved for training. Other advantages include fewer problems in getting permission to go on release courses, often closer contact with other trainees (very important for discussion of problems) and guaranteed quality control of posts.

The main disadvantage is that you may be stuck with a combination of posts you may not really like that much.

With the present difficulties in obtaining obstetric and paediatric senior house officer (SHO) posts if you are doing it yourself (see below) and the general benefit of not having to worry about new jobs for three years, most people now try and get on a vocational training scheme. Vacancies are advertised in the medical press, but information can also be obtained from regional postgraduate advisers and course organizers.

Do-it-yourself (DIY) schemes

These schemes may allow more flexibility in the location of the SHO jobs and in the type of jobs chosen. Trainees are sometimes forced to opt for DIY schemes if the vocational training scheme on offer does not contain the jobs that interest them.

DIY schemes also allow young doctors to keep their options open, if they are not yet certain which direction they want to take in medicine.

One common problem encountered in DIY schemes is convincing consultants that although you wish to be a GP you should still be allowed to fill their SHO post. Many specialists guard their posts jealously for doctors wishing to specialize in their branch of medicine.

Those on DIY schemes must also ensure that the post they wish to fill is educationally approved.

GUIDELINES FOR PROSPECTIVE TRAINEES

Selecting a course

There are many factors to be considered when selecting a vocational training scheme.

Location

If you particularly want to practise in one part of the country it is obviously desirable to find a training scheme there – you can then get to know the local GPs and they can get to know you. Getting a place is not, however, a guarantee of finding a permanent post in that area.

Content

Preferences as to content of the course are up to the individual, and unfortunately these cannot always be catered for. It is, however, best to have some obstetric experience somewhere in the scheme.

Some vocational training schemes begin with a three-month 'taster' of general practice and finish with the remaining nine months. Although unnerving, this combination can alert you to the important aspects of general practice that need to be learned in the subsequent hospital posts. Many trainees realize too late that they have not gained all they could have from their hospital jobs.

Some schemes contain posts which are far busier than others, similarly some entail the trainee doing a lot more on-call work. This is something of a two-edged sword, since busy jobs tend to mean you learn a lot, but equally you may not want to be continually exhausted. Check on this at the outset.

One of the best ways of finding out about a vocational training scheme is by talking to someone who is on one at the moment.

Selecting a training practice

Selecting a training practice can be a hazardous procedure. Although you only have to spend at most a year there, if it is unpleasant that year can be quite traumatic.

Find out as much as you can about the practice – talk to the present trainee.

Ask about how much teaching goes on, what the workload is like (this should not exceed that of the trainer) and about the on-call duties. The trainee is meant to be supernumerary and therefore surplus to requirements, the practice should not depend on the trainee to carry on its normal activities.

Ask about how easy it is to go off on release courses, how interested the other partners are and so on.

At best, the practice should provide a balance between good on-the-job experience and experience gained through direct teaching, and out of the practice visits (to the pharmacy, other practices, etc.).

Finally, do not go into a training practice expecting to find permanent employment. Even if a position does become available the partners are likely to advertise it before making a decision.

Trainers

Defining what makes a good or bad trainer can be difficult. As mentioned above, trainers have had to go through a fairly rigorous selection process to do the job, thus it must be assumed that in most cases they have the necessary skills to perform it. And they are also continually assessed by the regional advisers, through trainee reports filled in after finishing their in-practice experience, through assessment of the trainees performance on day-release courses and by the JCPTGP visitors.

Nevertheless, poor trainers do exist.

In the final analysis good trainers are those who do their job and try to instruct their trainees on how to be competent GPs. There are times when interpersonal problems obscure the abilities of a trainer, but a trainer is not necessarily 'bad' just because you do not get on.

Good trainers, should be giving you regular teaching, should be available to answer questions and should be supportive.

TRAINEES' PROBLEMS AND HOW TO DEAL WITH THEM

Training standards

It may be difficult to assess the standard of training you are receiving since you have no previous experience to compare it with. The best way to judge is to ask fellow trainees at the day release courses about what and how they are learning and if possible arrange a few visits to other practices.

If you are unhappy talk to your trainer first (do not immediately go above his head as this may complicate what may be an easily remediable problem). If, however, you have no success in improving things then talk to your course organizer and he will informally try and sort things out. If this still does not produce results then contact the regional adviser. It is not unknown for trainers to be removed from their position as a result of poor performance.

Contracts

It is still not the norm for all trainees to have a contract, but you would be strongly advised to have one. The British Medical Association (BMA) can provide specimen trainee contracts and if your trainer does not offer you one then suggest he adopts this.

Beware of contracts which are very different from the BMA's. A bad contract is worse than no contract at all.

Pay, expenses and conditions

Financially, you have a number of rights as a trainee and it is advisable (although boring) to have a good look at the relevant sections of the Red Book in order to be sure what they are. Your trainer, for instance, is obliged to provide you with on-call accommodation (the cost of which he can reclaim from the Family Practitioner Committee (FPC)) so do not be fobbed off with having to provide it for yourself if you do not need to.

Your pay and expenses are dealt with directly by the FPC. If you have any query give them a ring and ask. If you are confused your trainer or course organizer will usually be able to help.

Part Three
Practice Organization

Chapter 6

The NHS and the GP

The NHS is arbitrarily divided into two administrative parts. One is mostly concerned with primary care and the other with secondary care. However, there is considerable overlapping of some services.

FAMILY PRACTITIONER COMMITTEES

Family Practitioner Committees (FPCs) are now independent authorities and they administer and have contracts with general medical practitioners, general dental practitioners, chemists and opticians. They make sure that terms of service are complied with and they are responsible for making payments and monitoring standards.

Though working almost exclusively for the NHS, GPs are self employed. They contract with the FPC to 'provide all necessary medical services' and they are responsible for this all day and every day. These are onerous terms of service, as legally the GP is responsible for making sure that the patient gets any necessary care and when resources are scarce this is not always easy.

DISTRICT HEALTH AUTHORITIES

Secondary care is largely provided by District Health Authorities (DHAs) though they are also concerned with primary care because they are responsible for providing district nurses, health centres, health visitors and all the other community medical services. With an increasing emphasis on community care the influence of the hospitals on primary care is increasing.

REGIONAL HEALTH AUTHORITIES

Regional Health Authorities (RHAs) administer several DHAs and are responsible for providing regional special services such as neurosurgery. In their turn RHAs are responsible to the NHS Management Board and the DHSS.

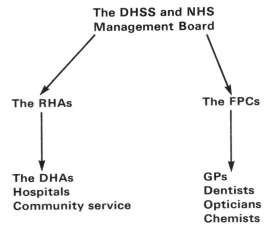

Figure 6.1

FINANCE

The FPCs services are not yet cash limited. This means that there is no theoretical limit to the money that can be spent. In reality, the GP's scope for earning fees is relatively limited though prescribing can be costly.

All the other NHS services are cash limited hence the waiting lists for hospital care and the increasing frustration in hospital doctors.

GPs can influence these authorities through their representatives who are members. All authorities are obliged to have GP members.

REMUNERATION

Details are in the Statement of Fees and Allowances, the Red Book issued by the DHSS containing all regulations and scales of payment for doctors. Make sure you read it.

- *Salary* is related to the last NHS hospital post held. Payment is increased on the incremental date to next point in the scale.
- *Removal expenses* may be paid. If in doubt contact the finance officer at the FPC.

- *Other earnings.* By regulation, the trainer cannot make any extra payments.
- *All fees* normally belong to the practice.
- *Part-time work* in off-duty hours. To do this, you must get the permission of the trainer *and the FPC*.
- *Telephone.* The cost of installing a new telephone or a bedside extension is reimbursable by the FPC.
- *Car allowance* is not automatically tax deductible and must be declared to the tax inspector.
- *Excess rent.* Look up in the Red Book or ask the FPC for details.
- *Interview expenses.* Expenses for an interview with a trainer are payable by the responsible FPC provided that an offered job is not refused without good reason.
- *Sickness.* Salary will be paid for up to three months. If the trainee is away for more than two weeks the training period will be extended to compensate for this.
- *Maternity leave.* To be eligible, the trainee must have completed at least 12 months of NHS service immediately before the application. For details see the Red Book.

Chapter 7

Medical records

The GP NHS medical records are unique in that they provide a life-long account of the patient's medical history. Virtually all the present stock of records are in the old Lloyd George envelopes because only a few GPs have been able to convert to A4-size records. The potential usefulness of the records as a clinical, teaching or research tool is often marred by the fact that information, if recorded at all, may be haphazard or illegible. Information retrieval is often laborious or impossible.

REASONS FOR GOOD RECORD-KEEPING

- To refresh your memory about your patient's history.
- To help other doctors who may see your patient.
- For medicolegal purposes.
- Research projects need accurate clinical information.
- Good records are useful tools in teaching sessions.
- Almost any audit process depends on accurate notes.

CHARACTERISTICS OF GOOD RECORDS

1 All episodes are recorded legibly.
2 Ideally each episode should have the following recorded:
   S (subjective)   Patients complaints and observations.
   O (objective)   Examination and investigations.
   A (analysis)   Concise summary of position.
   P (plan)   Plan of action.
3 Records should contain a data base with information about family history, past and present problems, social history, allergies, immunization status, etc.
4 The necessary information is easily retrievable.

HOW TO ACHIEVE GOOD RECORDS

- All hospital letters and continuation cards should be secured in chronological order.
- Use a standard format for recording episodes. You can use the mnemonic given above (that is SOAP) or invent your own.
- The data base. Make a point of recording occupation, marital status, etc., on the envelope. Some doctors keep the back of the envelope for notes on immunization and other indices. Some practices have a special data base card which can be filled in bit by bit or patients can be asked to fill in a questionnaire—easiest when they first join the practice.
- Once the volume of a record envelope gets beyond a certain point it becomes progressively more difficult to extract information quickly. A *summary* of major events on a separate card is helpful. Once this has been done the thick files may be filleted. Only the key letters and pathology forms need be retained.

RECORDS TO FACILITATE CONTINUOUS CARE

Most illnesses needing continuous care require the doctor to do routine checks, for example, diabetics should have their fundi looked at once a year. This process is made easier if special cards are used. The universally accepted example of this is the antenatal cooperation card. Similar cards have been designed for diabetes, hypertension and family planning.

Repeat prescribing may also be better controlled if patients on regular medication have their details recorded on special cards which also note the number of prescriptions issued and when the patient should be seen next.

RESEARCH REGISTERS

These are simply files of information about patients which allow easy abstraction of statistical and other information.

AGE–SEX REGISTER

The age–sex register is the basic register for any type of statistical research work. It can also be used to identify certain groups for surveillance, for example, cervical smears for women over 35.

DISEASE REGISTERS

These are lists of patients with certain illnesses. The numbers recorded will be as large or as small as the doctor's interests dictate. Useful as a quick way to identify groups of patients with certain illnesses for research, audit or teaching purposes.

THE A4 RECORD

A large file to take A4 sheets. Theoretically the larger format should help the doctor to maintain useful and tidy notes. However, the larger size does not ensure good records (remember what most hospital files look like).

Advantages

- More space for recording details.
- Larger format should make them tidier.
- Hospital letters and forms may be filed flat.

Disadvantages

- Can just become large untidy notes.
- More space needed—more cabinets—bigger rooms.
- Cost of conversion can be quite high.

FAMILY RECORDS

Some practices file all the records of the members of a family together. Useful if you wish to refer to the others during a consultation.

COMPUTERS

Computers are unintelligent machines which can store, recall and analyse data quickly and accurately. The principal difficulty in their use for GP records is the time and effort needed to get data into them in the first place.

Computers are good for:

- Age–sex registers.
- Disease registers.

- Repeat prescribing.
- Recall registers and screening programmes.
- Audit.
- Epidemiological research.
- Word processing.

Though it needs more effort, computers can also be used for:

- Event recording.
- Acute prescribing.

A practice should be well organized *before* getting a computer.

The small practice with good manual office systems has little need for a computer. The principal attraction would be the repeat prescribing systems.

CONFIDENTIALITY

The GP should make sure that his records remain confidential. They should be secure when not in use and the staff should be given access only on an essential-user basis.

Chapter 8

Certificates

Issuing certificates is an essential though not always enjoyable part of the GP's job. When you sign one you are putting the authority of your profession behind it. Never do this unless you are sure of the facts and that it is justified. You may often be pressed to give certificates without seeing the patient or on tenuous grounds. Do not give in to emotional or financial persuasion.

False certification is an offence that can be reported to the General Medical Council (GMC). In most years one or two doctors are disciplined for this – so beware.

NHS CERTIFICATES

The GP is obliged by his terms of service to issue certificates without payment to patients who are entitled to them.

Sickness

Patients in employment are entitled to certificates if they have been or are likely to be off work for a week or longer and if they are covered or have an industrial disease. For the first week off work they can use a self-certificate – this should not involve the doctor.

Form Med. 3

This is the usual certificate for sickness. It is used for insurance purposes only, and the patient must be seen. At the back of the pad there are forms for requesting the regional medical officer to give an opinion about the patient's fitness for work. You must also notify him if you have used a false diagnosis on the certificate.

Form Med. 5

This certificate is for use retrospectively or when the patient has not been seen but is under hospital care.

Maternity

These certificates enable expectant mothers to claim the various benefits to which they are entitled.

Form FW8

This is issued at the start of the pregnancy, enables mothers to claim free prescriptions, dental treatment, etc.

Mat. B1

This is issued after the 26th week and entitles mothers to a maternity grant and allowance.

PRIVATE CERTIFICATES

A doctor is not obliged to issue these. The BMA issues lists of recommended fees. Private certificates should not be issued any more casually than NHS ones.

REPORTS

Employers, insurance companies, solicitors and many other agencies may approach the GP for reports on patients.

1   Make sure the patient gives consent in writing or through an agent.
2   Draw the attention of the patient to any detrimental information you have before you make the report.
3   Remember patients have a right to see insurance reports if they so wish. If a patient has indicated that he wishes to read such a report before it is sent off the practice must keep it for him. In all cases a copy of such reports must be kept by the practice for 6 months.
4   Reports should go direct to another professional – a solicitor, for example.
5   Be sure of your facts. You may be questioned about them in court.

DEATH CERTIFICATES

It is a statutory obligation to issue a death certificate.

- Write clearly and make sure of your facts.
- There is no legal necessity to visit after death, but it is kind and advisable to do so.
- Do not issue a certificate if the patient was not seen within two weeks of death or if you have any doubt about the nature of the death (see page 156). Read the instructions in the front of the book of certificates.

CREMATION CERTIFICATES

Part I

This is normally given by the doctor issuing the death certificate. The body must be seen and examined.

Part II

This is given by an independent doctor of at least five years' standing who should question the patient's doctor and relatives or nurses. You must see and examine the body.

Chapter 9

The practice team

TEAM WORK

The practice team is a fine concept. GPs used to work in isolation (and some still do). There has been a progressive trend towards the development of group practices and the employment of ancillary staff such as secretaries and receptionists. In many areas primary care in the community is now a team effort.

There are advantages and disadvantages to team work.

Advantages

- Improving communication.
- Dissemination of knowledge.
- Maximum use of specialist skills.
- Sharing of responsibility.
- Understanding the work of others.

Disadvantages

- Personality clashes and status problems.
- Shelving or dodging responsibility.
- Patient may not know whom to relate to.
- A big team needs organization.
- Time needed for meetings.

COMPOSITION OF THE TEAM

1 The GPs and the staff employed by them.
2 Staff employed by the health authority.
3 Occasionally staff employed by other agencies, eg. social services.

HEALTH AUTHORITY STAFF

These are community workers who may cover a geographical area or who may be attached to a GP. They are primarily responsible to the health authority and GPs therefore have to work with them rather than over them:

- District nurses.
- Health visitors.
- Midwives.
- Specialized nurses, e.g. diabetic, incontinence, stoma, drug abuse, geriatric.
- Social workers.

District nurses

- They are state registered nurses (SRNs) usually with special training, who do home nursing.
- In some areas they are allowed to work in surgeries.
- They may be assisted by state enrolled nurses (SENs) or unqualified bath assistants.
- Good relationships are essential because the district nurse will be looking after most of the chronically sick patients in the practice.
- They are experts in obtaining sick room equipment, night care, and other aids.

Health visitors

- They are SRNs who also have at least part I of the midwifery certificate.
- Further training is necessary to obtain the health visitors' certificate.
- Their work is directed by the community nursing officer.
- They are obliged to visit all newborn babies as soon as possible after the midwife stops attending.
- A major part of their work is the supervision of children in the community. Regular assessment of developing children with the objective of detecting physical, social or mental handicaps takes up much of their time.
- They may also undertake health education, run relaxation and mothercraft classes, and give counselling to families with social and emotional difficulties.
- Mothers use health visitors for advice about all sorts of problems and some of their work overlaps that of social workers.

Community midwives

- Midwives are SRNs who go on to obtain parts I and II of the midwifery certificate.
- Their work includes making sure that home conditions are suitable for confinements or for early discharge from hospital; undertaking deliveries in the home or in GP obstetric units; and doing antenatal care either in the GP's surgery or on their own.

Specialized nurses

- There is an increasing tendency for district health authorities to train and deploy specialized nurses in the community.
- They can be valuable allies in the care of patients with particular problems.

Social workers

- Most social workers are in teams allocated to a geographical area. Very few are attached to GPs.
- Relationships are much better if you get to know your local social workers and make sure that they can contact you when necessary.
- Their main statutory duty is the supervision of the welfare of children in the community.
- They also undertake the community care of the mentally handicapped, the physically handicapped, the elderly, people with social or emotional problems, and the mentally ill.

STAFF EMPLOYED BY THE GP

Telephonists, receptionists and secretaries

In small practices the same staff may have to fulfil all these functions. In larger units they may specialize. Receptionists have a vital role in the practice. Usually they are the point of first contact, so a kind, efficient response from them is essential.

Receptionist work

The work of receptionists may include the following:

- *Appointments.* Keeping the doctor and the patients happy.

- *Visits.* Taking messages for home visits. Trying to match expectations of patients and views of the GP.
- *Prescriptions.* Taking messages and filling in the FP 10s as directed.
- *Forms.* Registering new patients. Dealing with claim forms for item-of-service fees.
- *Surgery.* Running surgery sessions smoothly. Keeping doctor to time tactfully.
- *Records.* Getting records in and out of the files. Tidying up records and filing letters.
- *Advice.* Giving simple advice about other services, welfare foods, clinics, etc.

Make sure that the staff doing a responsible job get adequate training and remuneration. Give clear instructions and regularly discuss problems with them.

The practice manager

Discovering the joys of delegation, more GPs are appointing managers. They may be full-time or part-time depending on the size of the practice and the work delegated.

The main functions are as follows:

- *Staff management.* Dealing with training, wages, tax and problems.
- *Stock control.* Obtaining drugs, dressings, stationery.
- *Maintenance.* Organizing cleaning, repairs, decorating.
- *The FPC.* Dealing with forms, claims, records.
- *Accounts.* Keeping the practice books.
- *Initial management* of patient complaints and problems.

Nurses

An increasing number of GPs are employing their own nurses because it is easier to direct their work and to make it fit in with the surgery hours. Most of them are employed in treatment rooms. Their functions are.

- Nursing procedures, dressings, injections.
- Dealing with pathology specimens, taking blood and urine samples.
- Handling stock control of drugs.

- Giving advice about simple illnesses.
- Assisting at minor operations, eg fitting intrauterine contraceptive devices.
- Undertaking electrocardiograms (ECGs).
- Undertaking immunization.

Some doctors are offering nurses of suitable calibre further training to extend the scope of their work. They may then undertake the following duties:

- Health screening.
- Routine follow-up of chronic illnesses such as hypertension, diabetes and obesity.
- Visiting the housebound.
- Family planning advice, repeat pills, caps.
- Cervical smears.
- First visits for simple illnesses like chickenpox.
- Special investigations, ECGs and allergy tests.
- Preconceptual advice.

Whatever role is delegated to nurses, GPs have the responsibility of ensuring that nurses are adequately trained and that they agree to the delegation.

Chapter 10

The GP as an employer

Like many other employers, the GP must comply with the Employment Acts. Employees must have proper job description, a contract, comfortable and safe conditions of work. National Insurance and tax deductions must be made. 70 per cent of the salaries of up to two full-time staff per partner may be reclaimed from the Family Practitioner Committee (FPC), claims being made each quarter on form ANC3.

HEALTH CENTRES

In most centres staff are employed direct by the health authority, 30 per cent of the cost then being reclaimed from the GPs (in a few health centres the GPs are allowed to hire their own staff).

Advantages

- GPs are relieved of the tasks of hiring and firing.
- There is no work concerned with wages, tax, etc.

Disadvantages

- Staff are tied to pay scales that are sometimes inadequate.
- The system is often inflexible.

THE GP MEMBERS OF THE TEAM

The GP is an independent business person who contracts with the FPC to provide a primary medical service for the patients on the practice list. As from the 16 August 1982 all principals entering general practice will have to be vocationally trained for three years or to have had equivalent experience approved by the Joint Committee for Postgraduate Training in General Practice (JCPTGP; see also Chapter 5).

A suitably trained doctor may enter practice in the following three ways:

1 By joining an established partnership.
2 By applying for a vacancy advertised by a FPC.
3 By setting up in practice in an open or a designated area. In a designated area an initial practice allowance may be payable.

Finance

The practice is paid a basic practice allowance for each partner. Capitation and item of service fees are then added as appropriate.

There are special allowances for seniority, vocational training and designated areas. All the details are in the Statement of Fees and Allowances (SFA); make sure you get a copy and read it.

Partners divide the income according to the practice agreement. The only regulation is that the lowest paid partner must not earn less than one-third the share of the highest paid one.

Contracts

Like any other business arrangement the partnership should be regulated by a carefully drafted contract. The characteristics of a good partnership are:

- There should be an equitable distribution of income.
- Adequate provision should be made for sickness, maternity leave, etc.
- Decisions should be taken democratically.
- Partners should be encouraged to develop new ideas and interests.
- Regular meetings should be held to discuss administration and clinical practice.

Assistants

Some practices employ an assistant rather than take on a new partner because:

- The relationship is that of employee to employer.
- The FPC does make a payment for an assistant but this is less than the basic practice allowance for a partner.

Trainers

To be a trainer the GP has to be appointed by the GP subcommittee of the Regional Postgraduate Committee. The criteria for selection vary from region to region, but usually include:

- At least three years in practice.
- Good references.
- Premises, records and facilities must pass inspection by the regional adviser.
- Attendance at a trainer's course.
- Taking an active part in local workshops and postgraduate meetings.

Trainers have to submit themselves to reselection at regular intervals.

Locums

Locums are necessary in small practices to maintain a service during leave and sickness absences.

- The GP is responsible for finding locums and for making sure that they are competent.
- If the locum is in breach of the terms of service the GP is responsible.
- In certain circumstances the FPC will pay part of the cost of a locum.

Part Four
Relations with others in the practice

Chapter 11

In the practice

PATIENTS AND FAMILIES

In order to enjoy general practice as a way of life and achieve professional satisfaction and respect, it is essential to maintain a good long-term relationship with your patients. It takes a considerable amount of skill to remain friendly and approachable and yet maintain the degree of objectivity which is required for firm management in the patient's best interests. The essential features of a good doctor–patient relationship in general practice include the following.

Mutual respect

The patient must respect the doctor as a person and as a medical technician. However it is up to the doctor to merit that respect and not assume it.

The doctor must recognize the fact that every patient has an individual importance and dignity and a life of their own to lead. Remember that your patients provide you with your living.

Confidentiality

Confidentiality is vital. The patient must be able to rely on the doctor's discretion. Unless there are compelling reasons for doing so, information must not be disclosed to anyone else, including close relatives, without the patient's permission. Adolescents sometimes present a particular problem in this respect.

Generally accepted reasons for breaking such confidence include:

- Telling close relatives about a serious diagnosis like cancer, when it may be necessary to plan appropriate care.
- Where the rights of the community override those of the individual, e.g. the engine driver who develops epilepsy. Even in these cases the patient should be informed of the doctor's proposed course of action. If in doubt, consult your defence organization.

Willingness to give a good service

A practice which tries to provide a good service will benefit greatly from enhanced doctor–patient relationships. The patient who regards his/her doctor as well intentioned is much more likely to accept their opinion about what is appropriate in terms of treatment, referral or home visiting.

Sensitivity

In order to be successful and function well as a personal doctor it is necessary to make a conscious effort to understand your patients' feelings and the way they think. Dealing with symptoms at a superficial level can make life easier and consultations quicker in the short term, but you are likely to miss the real reasons for the consultation and impair your ability to treat the whole person.

- Concentrate on listening rather than talking.
- 'Open' questions allow patients more scope for expressing themselves than 'closed' questions, e.g. 'How do you feel?' gives the patient more scope than: 'Do you feel tense?', which invites a monosyllabic answer.

Honesty

In any healthy relationship both parties should be as honest as possible with each other. Very often it is the doctor's emotions, and his/her inability to handle them which prevent an honest exchange and communication may break down. Patients may feel isolated and rejected if they think that the truth is being withheld.

The skill in handling these problems lies in being able to determine how much the patient really wants to know. A nonspecific question like: 'What do you know about your illness?' gives the patient an opportunity to ask for more information. In general, specific questions from patients should be given honest replies.

Responsibility

It is your professional duty to help your patients appropriately and to the best of your ability. This does not mean that you have to respond to frivolous applications for housing transfers, and certainly not to comply with totally inappropriate or even illegal requests, but it does mean that you may have to spend time and energy trying to solve real problems.

Referral to a consultant does not mean relinquishing responsibility. If the advice on management seems to you to be unhelpful or wrong, then you must say so and take appropriate action. Sometimes relatives or other professionals may urge you to embark on a course of action which you may feel is not in the best interests of your patient, e.g. admitting an elderly, mildly confused lady into hospital. If you think that it would be kinder to keep her at home, and you are prepared to provide the necessary services, then you should do so – the patient's interests are paramount.

PARTNERS AND COLLEAGUES

Partners

A practice cannot function properly if the partners are at loggerheads. A few guidelines may be helpful:

- Partners must be carefully chosen to be compatible.
- A good and fair contract is essential.
- Work and income must be shared equitably.
- Decision-making must be democratic.
- Regular meetings should be held and minutes kept.
- Basic clinical and administrative policies should be agreed and respected by all partners.

Neighbours

Friction with neighbouring colleagues is much less likely if you get to know them socially and professionally.

Do not agree to see patients of your colleagues without permission, except in an emergency. This also applies to private patients.

If you are in an out-of-hours rota make sure that you find out how the others like to manage their patients. Never make overt or implied criticisms of your colleagues' treatment. Some patients are very skilful at playing one doctor off against another. Careful notes must be kept and forwarded to the patient's regular doctor. Never forget the value of the telephone.

Primary care team

Most practices now employ practice nurses and work in association with community nurses and health visitors. An increasing number have attached community psychiatric nurses, clinical psychologists and social workers and almost all employ several clerical and administrative staff.

Relationships are likely to be enhanced if a few simple guidelines are followed:

- Fellow professionals should be treated as highly trained colleagues with their own fund of experience and expertise.
- Remember that they usually work in an hierarchical structure and are accountable to their superiors in a way that you are not. Sometimes this may conflict with their loyalties and responsibilities to the team.
- The best way of ironing out problems, avoiding manipulation by patients or clients, and providing the optimum service for them is to meet on a regular basis and to attend case-conferences whenever possible.
- Good teamwork takes time and effort but this is amply repaid by professional satisfaction and mutual support.

Private practice

Regulations

- You cannot charge your NHS patients for any *medical* service even if, in your view, it is outside the normal range of services.
- You can charge for private certificates, private prescriptions and medical examinations for employment, insurance and driving purposes.

Ethics

Remember that the patients who do come to see you privately may well be on someone else's NHS list and it is wise to ask your colleague's permission and find out about current treatment.

Insurance reports

Once a patient has authorized the insurance company to obtain a report you must provide an honest account of the facts. It would be reasonable, however, to make sure that your patient is fully aware of any significant information which might have to be included if the report was to be completed, e.g. the results of any tests for HIV (human immunodeficiency virus) infection.

If examination is requested then this will take at least 20 minutes and time should be set aside at the end of surgery or at a separate session.

Chapter 12

Hospitals

The hospital provides a variety of support services for the GP including beds, specialist opinions, concentrated nursing care, an accident and emergency department, physiotherapy and occupational therapy, x-ray and pathology services and a postgraduate education centre.

ACUTE ADMISSIONS

Acute admissions are usually arranged through the junior staff of the appropriate department by telephone. In case of difficulty do not hesitate to contact the responsible consultant.

THE ACCIDENT AND EMERGENCY DEPARTMENT

The accident and emergency (A&E) department should ideally be used, as the name implies, only for accidents and emergencies. However, some patients, especially in large towns and cities, regularly use these departments as an inappropriate alternative source of primary care and sometimes for the purpose of gaining a second opinion on their condition. GPs can help by educating their patients about the proper use of these facilities, providing reliable out-of-hours cover and making their own referrals to these departments appropriate.

REFERRALS (see also pages 123, 124)

In any one year 15 to 20 per cent of people in the UK are referred by their GP to a consultant for a specialist opinion and/or technical expertise.

Whenever there is a choice, consideration should always be given to the consultant's personality, interests and special expertise in relation to the patient and his/her particular problem.

On average, a GP will write eight referral letters a week and the best ones will be brief and to the point explaining the nature of the problem, detailing what investigations and treatment have been carried out, explaining why the referral is taking place and outlining what is expected from the consultant.

A cardinal ethical rule is that no consultant should see a patient without a referral letter from a GP. This still holds true for NHS patients although, unfortunately, some consultants seem prepared to give their opinion to unreferred patients prepared to pay for the privilege.

If there is a long waiting list for an outpatient appointment or for an operation then the GP may need to consider alternative strategies:

- The referral may be for a minor condition in which delay will do no harm.
- The patient may wish to consider a private referral or referral to another hospital.
- The patient may be encouraged to keep in close touch with the consultant's secretary in order to take advantage of a cancellation.
- If the condition of the patient warrants it, the GP may choose to contact the consultant personally, by letter or telephone, in order to press the patient's case.
- If the patient is still unsatisfied he/she should be advised to complain directly to the hospital administrator and to the local Member of Parliament, since the provision of adequate resources is, ultimately, a political decision.

The responsibility of the GP is to refer a patient when he/she is not able to provide the investigation, treatment or care which the patient requires. However, occasionally a patient may request a second opinion when this seems inappropriate or unnecessary and the doctor may feel upset, bewildered, rejected or even angry. In this situation the reasons for the patient's request should be calmly explored:

- Is the patient unhappy with the care provided so far? If so, in what way?
- Does the patient not believe or accept the diagnosis?
- Are the implications of the diagnosis so serious that a second opinion is desirable?
- Does the patient, or his relatives, feel that alternative or better treatment is available elsewhere?

Further discussion is likely to result in one of the following outcomes:

- The patient's fears or worries may be allayed and the doctor–patient relationship enhanced.
- The doctor may be helped to improve the standard of care or, at least, the patient's perception of it.
- A reasonable referral may be instituted without acrimony, either NHS or privately.
- A totally unreasonable or inappropriate request may be turned down after careful consideration and explanation.
- On occasion, there may be a recognition that the doctor–patient relationship has broken down and that it would be best for the patient to see a different doctor.

A few patients constantly seek second opinions, without paying much attention to the first, and this pattern of behaviour should be recognized and pointed out to the patient.

PATHOLOGY AND IMAGING FACILITIES

There are some fundamental differences between general practice and hospital medicine which affect the use of these departments considerably:

- Many illnesses seen by the GP are minor and self-limiting, thus investigation may be of no value in guiding treatment and the patient may well have recovered before the results become available.
- Many GPs are some distance from the nearest hospital. Special arrangements must therefore be made to transport specimens to the laboratory or the patient may have to travel,to the department at considerable expense and inconvenience.
- Over 90 per cent of all episodes of illness are managed entirely in primary care. The investigative services would soon be over-loaded if GPs were not selective in their use.

Nevertheless, selective and judicious use of open access to these hospital facilities enables the GP to investigate and manage many patients himself, thus increasing his own job satisfaction, reducing the load on out patient departments and saving patients both time and expense.

When requesting investigations consider the following criteria:

- Is this investigation necessary in order to clinch an important diagnosis, e.g. a mid-stream urine in a suspected urinary tract infection in a small child?
- Is this investigation necessary in order to exclude serious disease, e.g. an erythrocyte sedimentation rate in suspected temporal arteritis or a chest x-ray where carcinoma of the lung is a possibility?
- Might the results of this investigation lead to a change in treatment, e.g. finding trichomonas in a high vaginal swab?
- Will the inconvenience to the patient and the cost of the procedure be justified in relation to the value of the results obtained, e.g. a barium meal for vague dyspepsia of short duration?
- Are there any special features of the investigation which require the patient to be provided with prior detailed instructions, e.g. overnight fasting before lipoprotein estimation? If in doubt, look it up or telephone the department for advice.
- Can the specimen be delivered to the laboratory at a suitable time for them to process it, e.g. reliable estimations of serum potassium cannot be performed on an old specimen of blood.
- Is the patient on any medication which might affect the results of the investigation, e.g. antibiotics when bacteriological swabs are taken?
- Is the patient very young, very old, pregnant or suffering from any other condition which might affect the results?
- Is the patient at any risk from this investigation, e.g. x-rays in women of child-bearing age?

Whenever embarking on investigations treat the request as a consultation with a colleague, not as an order to a technician. Most consultant pathologists and radiologists are only too happy to give advice on appropriate tests or specific investigations required in a particular case and to clarify the significance of the results obtained.

Chapter 13

Local services

REGISTRAR OF BIRTHS AND DEATHS

Part of the registrar's job is to monitor the issuing of death certificates and he/she cannot register a death if the certificate is unsatisfactory in any way.

Certified procedure

- Avoid delay in issuing the certificate.
- The certificate is usually taken to the registrar by the relatives, but it is the doctor's responsibility to make sure that it gets there.
- Use legible handwriting or block capitals.
- Make sure the diagnosis is compatible with the International Classification of Diseases.
- *Do not* issue a certificate if you have any suspicion that the death was not natural.

If the body is to be cremated then it is necessary to complete an additional form, the second part of which must also be completed by an experienced doctor who has been fully registered for at least five years. The undertaker will provide the appropriate form and a fee is payable.

THE CORONER

Normally you should communicate with the coroner through his/her officer. The easiest way to establish contact is to telephone the local police station.

Reasons for reporting a death:

- Sudden, unexplained or unexpected death or where the doctor has not attended within 14 days.
- Unnatural abortion.
- Where accidents or injuries have contributed to death.

- Where there were industrial diseases or war pensioners' injuries present.
- Death after anaesthetic or operation.
- Where there were drug mishaps or abuse, alcoholism or poisoning.
- Where persons were in legal custody.
- Stillbirth after 24 weeks.
- Where there is any suspicion of crime or suicide.

When in doubt always err on the side of reporting the death. Very often the coroner will authorize you to issue a certificate if you are sure that the cause of death was a natural one.

POLICE AND POLICE SURGEONS

The police are normally very helpful to doctors and are prepared to provide an escort if the doctor has grounds to suspect that a patient may be violent or deranged. They will also help in the admission to hospital of a patient sectioned under the Mental Health Act. However, in the course of over-zealous investigation they may sometimes request confidential information in respect of a patient. You should be extremely cautious in providing such information without the patient's knowledge and it is usually best to check with your defence organization.

Police surgeons are doctors, often GPs who are contracted to provide a service to the police. They are becoming increasingly professional and most have had special training for their duties. As a rule it is better to leave all forensic work, e.g. suspected rape, assault or murder, to them rather than to meddle inappropriately.

SCHOOL HEALTH SERVICES

The district community health physician is responsible for the school health service including pre-school health checks by medical officers, advice regarding educational provision for handicapped children and the school nursing service. However, GPs and health visitors inevitably develop links with their local schools.

Teachers are in contact with children all day and can often provide a good assessment of the physical and emotional state of a child. Some teachers have special training in counselling techniques and many secondary schools have a welfare officer who often becomes involved with family problems as a consequence of his/her role in investigating non-attendance.

Children with infectious diseases must be excluded from school and home tuition may be available during the course of a long illness. Teachers may also need advice on the provision of medication, e.g. anticonvulsants or inhalers used by children before physical activities.

CHILD GUIDANCE CLINICS

These clinics are hybrids, funded by the District Health Authority (DHA) and the Local Education Authority (LEA). They deal with emotional problems in children under the age of 14 years, which are very commonly due to family dysfunction.

Referral may be made by GPs or by the educational psychologist employed by the LEA. Most clinics are orientated towards family therapy under the direction of a team consisting of social workers, psychologists and child psychiatrists.

SOCIAL SERVICES

Social services departments are financed and administered by the local authority and are quite separate from the health services. Their principal responsibilities are set out below:

- *Children.* Supervising the care of children in the community, identifying those at risk, taking them into care if necessary. Supervising fostering and adoption.
- *Elderly.* Supervising the care of the elderly in the community. Providing home care services (home helps) and homes for the elderly.
- *Handicapped.* Supervising the care of the physically and mentally handicapped. Providing aids, housing adaptations and sheltered workshops.
- *Mentally ill.* Providing community care and hostel accommodation. Making applications for compulsory admission to hospital under the Mental Health Act.
- *Families.* The caring of families in financial, social or emotional trouble, giving advice, counselling and welfare rights information.

Since only a minority of social workers are attached to primary health care teams it can be difficult to maintain good communications.

Cooperation is enhanced by having regular meetings and by each having easy access to the other. Understanding each others training, responsibilities, abilities and limitations will make referral more effective and relevant.

FAMILY PLANNING CLINICS

Family planning clinics were originally established and run as charities, but are now financed by the DHA. Patients may attend without referral, but most clinics are careful to inform the GP about advice given and contraceptives prescribed. If the GP is asked if there are any contraindications to using the pill it is the GP's responsibility to check up on this and to reply if necessary.

PREGNANCY ADVICE CENTRES

Pregnancy counselling clinics now exist in every large city. Some are charitable foundations which charge modest fees but many are purely commercial. They will usually see patients with or without a referral letter and their interpretation of the abortion law is liberal.

MARRIAGE GUIDANCE

There are two major charitable agencies which provide this service, one is non-denominational and the other Catholic. Carefully selected and highly trained counsellors provide a service which, in some centres, includes sex therapy.

VOLUNTARY SERVICES

There is a vast range of local and national services available. Social services or the local council offices are the best source of information and lists are also published from time to time in the medical press. Some of the best known include:

- *Samaritans.* An emergency contact for emotionally upset people.
- *Cruse.* A support service for the bereaved.
- *Citizen's Advice Bureaux.* Give advice about legal and welfare rights problems.
- *Grapevine.* Counselling for young people.

- *Old People's Welfare*. Arrange clubs, outings, meals and social activities for the elderly.
- *Alcoholics Anonymous*. Provide counselling and group support for people who wish to overcome dependence on alcohol.

SCREENING

The number of screening services available in the private sector is increasing, and it is fashionable for firms to finance this service for their executives. The ritual is elaborate, expensive and of doubtful value but reports are submitted to the patient's GP and occasionally provide a useful basis for health education.

EMPLOYMENT MEDICAL SERVICES

A few large commercial organizations employ their own full-time industrial medical officers, but most smaller concerns employ local GPs on a sessional basis.

The type and conditions of work can affect the health of your patients in a variety of ways. Make an effort to look around local factories so that you get to know more about working conditions. You can improve patient care by:

- Making a note of the patient's occupation on the records.
- Asking about hazards at work.
- Giving advice about how to minimize risks, e.g. teaching a patient with back trouble how to lift a heavy object.
- Contacting the factory doctor if working conditions need to be modified.
- Responding promptly to requests for information from the factory doctor, providing always that you have the patient's written permission.

REGIONAL MEDICAL OFFICERS

Regional medical officers (RMOs) are employed by the DHSS in order to monitor sickness certification and prescribing. In addition, they are available for help and advice on any aspect of practice including accommodation and buildings.

DRUG COMPANIES AND REPRESENTATIVES

The medical profession has an ambivalent relationship with the pharmaceutical industry. On the one hand, we tend to be suspicious of the commercial orientation of the companies but, on the other, most of us accept hospitality at postgraduate meetings and all of us read journals which are largely supported by advertising. A few guidelines might be of help:

- Decide whether you wish to see representatives in the practice or not and stick to your decision.
- If you do see representatives treat them courteously but treat their information critically.
- Be very suspicious of spurious 'drug trials' which are, in fact, thinly disguised marketing exercises, particularly if the payment offered is excessive for the work undertaken.
- Remember that, as a rule, it is best to use a small number of drugs regularly and only change your prescribing habits when there is clear evidence of a better alternative.

FAMILY PRACTITIONER COMMITTEES

The local Family Practitioner Committee (FPC) is most important for the GP. It is the contracting body which pays and administers general practice. Trainees should make a point of visiting the FPC and meeting the administrator and his/her colleagues.

Chapter 14

National professional organizations

THE GENERAL MEDICAL COUNCIL

The General Medical Council (GMC) was set up in 1858 and is a statutory body responsible directly to the Privy Council. Its chief function is to keep the medical register and the other roles stem from this major responsibility. All medical practitioners must be registered with the GMC and an annual retention fee is payable.

The medical register

Doctors may be granted provisional, limited or full registration.

Education

The GMC is responsible for monitoring standards of undergraduate education and is taking an increasing interest in postgraduate training.

Overseas doctors

The GMC is responsible for ensuring that overseas qualifications are commensurate with those in the UK.

Professional conduct

There are no set rules but case law has been developed as to what constitutes 'serious professional misconduct'. About a thousand complaints about doctors are made each year of which some 30 to 40 reach public hearings.

The type of serious professional misconduct in order of frequency are as follows:

- Abuse of alcohol or drugs.
- Theft, fraud or dishonesty.

- Disregard of care of patients.
- Canvassing and advertising.
- Improper relationships with patients (sexual or otherwise).
- Indecency.

Sick doctors

A new health committee is now able to deal with sick doctors without them having to appear in public. An alternative informal service is provided by the National Counselling Service for Sick Doctors (tel: 01 580 3160), which provides support and counselling services by national advisers. These are experienced doctors, drawn from every specialty including general practice, who work in a voluntary capacity.

BRITISH MEDICAL ASSOCIATION

About 70 per cent of the medical profession are members of the British Medical Association (BMA) and it is the principal medicopolitical body for doctors, although smaller groups such as the Medical Practitioners Union (MPU), the Socialist Medical Association (SMA) and the Conservative Medical Association (CMA) are also active.

The BMA:

- Negotiates with the Government on pay and conditions of work in the NHS.
- Provides advice and guidance on many general and personal professional matters.
- Publishes the *British Medical Journal* (*BMJ*) and other journals and books.
- Organizes national and local medicopolitical and social activities.
- Provides membership of most important governmental and professional committees.

GENERAL MEDICAL SERVICES COMMITTEE

The General Medical Services Committee (GMSC) is really a subcommittee of the BMA, but it includes representatives of non-members so that it is able to represent all GPs in the UK. It negotiates pay and conditions of work with the government on behalf of all NHS GPs .

LOCAL MEDICAL COMMITTEES

The Local Medical Committee (LMC) is elected by all GPs in a locality to represent their views to the Family Practitioner Committee (FPC) and other NHS bodies. Trainees elect their own representative to the LMC.

Representatives of LMCs meet in an annual conference which shapes national policy about general practice matters and guides the negotiations of the GMSC.

ROYAL COLLEGE OF GENERAL PRACTITIONERS

The Royal College of General Practitioners (RCGP) was founded in 1952 as the academic voice and image of general practice. Over half of all GPs are now members or fellows. Admission is by examination, although associate membership is open to all. The major activities of the college include:

- Conducting the MRCGP examination twice a year. Nearly 2000 candidates take the examination each year and the pass rate is about 70 per cent.
- Publishing the college journal (*JRCGP*) and numerous reports and papers.
- Organizing research and advising individuals embarking on research projects.
- Organizing local activities at faculty level and national activities and conferences.
- Supervising vocational training via its representatives on the JCPTGP (see page 19).

MEDICAL DEFENCE ORGANIZATIONS

Although membership is not compulsory in law it is essential that any doctor in practice, including a trainee, joins an approved medical defence organization, e.g. Medical Defence Union, Medical Protection Society, and Medical and Dental Defence Union of Scotland.

Defence organizations provide:

- Medicolegal advice and support.
- Legal representation at courts and inquiries.
- Financial indemnities for professional claims.

Claims have increased sharply in recent years and, as a consequence, premiums are now over £1,000 per annum.

ROYAL SOCIETY OF MEDICINE

Although the Royal Society of Medicine (RSM) is based in London, membership is open to all doctors and the society provides educational and library services, accommodation, catering and social facilities in a club atmosphere. It has had a Section of General Practice since 1950.

Part Five
The Law and Behaviour

Chapter 15

Possible problems

GENERAL MEDICAL COUNCIL

All medical practitioners have to be fully registered with the General Medical Council (GMC) to be recognized and able to practise as GPs.

Note: Always notify the GMC of your correct address – an incorrect address can lead to the removal of a doctor's name from the medical register.

On registration each doctor is given a 'blue book' – *Professional Conduct and Discipline: Fitness to Practise* (*latest edition* 1987). This is the basis for conduct by doctors. Read it and keep it for reference.

MEDICAL DEFENCE ORGANIZATIONS

Always contact and seek advice from your defence organizations whenever there are problems that may involve you in any professional legal or possible disciplinary, procedures. A phone call will obtain expert advice, support and reassurance. Do not reply or report in such cases without their advice.

'NEGLECT OR DISREGARD OF PERSONAL RESPONSIBILITIES TO PATIENTS FOR THEIR CARE AND TREATMENT' (Blue Book)

Most complaints from patients are under this category, for example:
- Failure to visit a patient at home when requested.
- Failure to provide or arrange for treatment when necessary, i.e. failure to carry out proper examination or to refer to a specialist.

INAPPROPRIATE DELEGATION OF MEDICAL DUTIES TO PROFESSIONAL COLLEAGUES AND NURSES

This includes:

- Misuse of deputizing services.
- Asking nurses to undertake tasks for which they are untrained.

ABUSE OF PROFESSIONAL PRIVILEGES

- Prescribing is part of statutory duty of GP services but prescribing has to be with care and knowledge of possible risks and side effects.
- Prescription of drugs of dependence has to be with care and a register must be kept of scheduled drugs obtained by the GP and such drugs must be kept in a locked receptacle.
- Care must be taken in prescribing drugs for addicts and their names have to be notified to the Chief Medical Officer at the Home Office or equivalent body.
- Take care in prescribing for friends or relatives who may be under care of their own GP.

PERSONAL BEHAVIOUR

- Never, never drink and drive because all such convictions are reported to the GMC and action is always taken.
- Beware of taking drugs, prescribed and non-prescribed.
- Do not enter into emotional or sexual relationships with a patient (or with a member of a patient's family).
- Do not become involved in improper financial transactions within the NHS or outside, i.e. fraud, charging NHS patients fees.
- Do not act violently or indecently.
- Do not canvass patients, advertise or disparage colleagues.
- Take care in receiving gifts, loans or excessive hospitality from drug companies.
- Ownership or shares in nursing homes, etc. may cause problems – get legal advice.

CONFIDENTIALITY

Confidentiality is fundamental to a good doctor–patient relationship.
- Beware of loose talk within the practice or outside among friends or family.
- Do not provide any professional information to anyone without the patient's written permission – to relatives, friends, employees, solicitors, insurance companies.
- Exceptions are certain circumstances where safety of the community overrides the individual's right of confidentiality.

CONSENT

In general, a patient must give informed consent before any investigation or therapeutic treatment is carried out.

- Below the age of 16 the doctor must take care to balance the child's right to confidentiality with parental responsibilities and family stability. In particular, he/she has to decide on the child's maturity and ability to understand and appreciate – this applies particularly to prescribing contraceptives and in termination of pregnancy.
- Take special care in obtaining consent for participation in drug trials, provision of reports, autopsies (permission from family) and use of organs for transplantation.

Termination of pregnancy

A GP must act as a counsellor and, if there are grounds for terminating a pregnancy, he/she should arrange for a referral to a hospital or clinic.

If a doctor has a conscientious objection to terminating a pregnancy, then the patient must be given the opportunity to seek another opinion.

COMPLAINTS

Complaints against a GP may be made in the following ways:

- To the *practice* where they will be dealt with informally.
- To the *Family Practitioner Committee* where they may be dealt with by the chairperson, by attempted conciliation or referral to

a hearing by the Medical Services Committee.
- To the *GMC* in case of possible serious professional misconduct.
- To the *Courts* where a civil action may ensue.

To repeat, in all such cases seek the advice of your professional defence organization.

GENERAL ADVICE

Trainees must never be afraid of seeking advice and assistance from more senior colleagues, and it is always best, if possible, to get this advice before the event than after it has happened.

Part Six
Management

Chapter 16

Principles of treatment

The essential principles of management in general practice are, wherever possible:

- Cure.
- Relief.
- Comfort.
- Prevention.
- Rehabilitation and maintenance of function.

Many patients seen by GPs do not need prescribed medication, either for the relief of symptoms or to treat disease. Nevertheless if patients are anxious or distressed GPs may feel the need to give a prescription as a token of their sympathy and their willingness to help. They may believe that this is what patients expect. They may feel that they lack the necessary time for a detailed explanation that would be needed if they were not to provide prescriptions.

Those patients who do need medication usually have to be left in charge of administering it. Its efficacy may depend on the appreciation of its importance combined with intelligent and conscientious interpretation of the GP's instructions.

It is therefore much more difficult in general practice than in hospital to use drugs in a completely logical way and special care is needed to ensure safe and sensible prescribing and administration.

It may be helpful to work out personal codes and practice protocols and formularies for prescribing. Something basic and simple, along the lines of the list below, would do to start with. More detail can then be added if necessary.

- Prescribe nothing unless there is a clear clinical indication for it, i.e. an expectation that it will materially alter the course of the illness or relieve suffering.
- Choose the cheapest satisfactory form of the drug available.

- If the clinical indication is for a placebo, make sure that it is both safe and cheap.
- Make sure the patient agrees to take the drug, understands what it is for, and how it should be taken.

The GP needs to bear in mind what a patient needs to know about any drug.

- How should the drug be given, i.e. by what route, how often, when in relation to meals, for how long? Is it a short course or should it be continued indefinitely?
- What effect is it likely to have on the illness, i.e. immediate cure, delayed cure, relief of symptoms (complete or partial), no obvious effect?
- Should the drug be continued after the condition appears to have resolved?
- If the drug is to be taken 'as required', exactly what is the indication for a dose? How often may it be repeated? What is the maximum total dose in 24 hours?
- What side effects are to be expected, are likely, are possible but nothing to worry about, should be reported to the doctor, should make me stop taking the drug?
- How important is it to take the drug? What will happen if it is not taken?

To practise efficient prescribing, GPs need to have a clear idea of the following:

- Why exactly has the patient come to see the GP? Is it because he is anxious about the meaning of a symptom (e.g. whether the headache is due to a brain tumour)? Is he simply seeking symptomatic relief? Does he want to discuss some other problem?
- What is the diagnosis? Is medication likely to be useless, helpful, important, essential?
- If infection is present, what is the most likely organism, what is it likely to be sensitive to, and would the patient recover without a drug?
- If medication is not indicated, does the patient understand why? What can he do for himself?
- If medication is important, e.g. in hypertension, does the patient share the GP's enthusiasm and agree to take the drug? Is he capable of remembering to take it regularly?

- If the timing of doses is important and individually variable, e.g. sodium cromoglycate in asthma, does the patient understand how the drug works and how to work out, for himself, when to take it?

This sounds time-consuming but it can be covered quite briefly and if the end-result is that people become better educated about drugs and the management of minor illness, fewer patients will attend the surgery for problems which they can deal with quite competently without the help of a doctor.

Chapter 17

Common clinical problems

The new trainee in general practice often has considerable difficulty in reorientating his/her clinical approach and thinking from that acquired in hospital.

GPs are often apologetic because they do not have the time to follow the routine which they were taught as students – a detailed history and examination followed by appropriate investigations. A little reflection, however, will show that the approach of the orthopaedic surgeon, for instance, is very different from that of the gynaecologist, while the ophthalmologist and the thoracic surgeon have little in common. Each has had to modify his/her approach to clinical medicine in the light of the specialist function. The GP is no exception.

The issue for the new entrant to general practice is, therefore, how to adapt his/her basic clinical approach in a way which is safe, effective and relevant for primary care. Statistically, we know that most conditions seen in primary care are minor and self-limiting, while many of the others are chronic and persistent. Major life-threatening conditions are uncommon but it is essential that they should not be overlooked. Unfortunately, there is often little or no difference between the early symptoms of a major condition and the definitive symptoms of a minor condition. A cough, for example, may signify anything from a minor respiratory infection to a carcinoma of the bronchus.

In the section which follows we have chosen some common presenting symptoms and suggested a clinical approach that seems appropriate and relevant in the context of primary care. In the end every GP has to devise his/her own approach but these suggestions provide a starting point for consideration.

Emergencies are dealt with in Chapter 19.

HEADACHE

There is a persistent myth, common among patients and even some doctors, that headache is a symptom of a raised blood pressure (BP).

With the exception of the very rare case of malignant hypertension there is no basis for this belief.

Common causes

- *Tension* with or without anxiety/depression. Usually described as a tight band or pressure on top of the head or pain and tenderness in the occipital region.
- *Migraine.* A diagnostic point is the recurrent, episodic nature of the headache. The classic triad of unilateral headache, associated with visual disturbances and nausea/vomiting is less common than partial syndromes, i.e. common migraine.
- *Toxic.* Caused by infections, drugs (remember overuse of ergotamine), and alcohol.
- *Secondary* to other conditions affecting the head and neck, e.g. sinusitis, cervical spondylosis, ocular conditions.

Less common causes

- *Temporal arteritis* in the elderly.
- *Meningitis.*
- *Raised intracranial pressure* due to tumours, subdural haematoma, subarachnoid haemorrhage.

Pitfalls

- Pain due to raised intracranial pressure may not be severe initially. Persistant headache or pain which is unusual in type or frequency for that patient should arouse suspicion.
- Subarachnoid haemorrhage may present as severe migraine.
- Elderly patients with temporal arteritis may complain only of vague pains – remember the association with polymyalgia rheumatica.
- Children with space-occupying lesions may suffer remarkably mild headaches. Vomiting may be appreciable but the periodic syndrome (p86) is much more common than brain tumours.

Approach

History

Establish the site, frequency and intensity of headache, and ask about any associated symptoms, e.g. visual disturbances, vomiting, and any precipitating and relieving factors.

Examination

Examine the head, neck and fundi, and take the BP (the patient expects this, and it provides an opportunity for screening).

Management

Manage as appropriate to the diagnosis. If you are not sure, there is no harm in waiting and reviewing the patient a few days later.

PAIN IN THE CHEST

This symptom causes considerable anxiety in patients, especially young or middle-aged men who are worried about heart disease.

Common causes

• *Musculoskeletal.*
  Trauma, muscular spasm due to anxiety.
  Viral myalgia (mild Bornholm-type illness)
  Cough causing local strain or fracture.
  Tender costal cartilages (Tietze's syndrome).
  Referred pain, often girdle distribution, due to disorders of the thoracic spine.
• *Infective.* More often discomfort or soreness rather than pain.
• *Herpes zoster.*

Less common causes

• *Cardiovascular.* Ischaemic cardiac pain, pericarditis, pulmonary embolus.

- *Respiratory.* Pleurisy, pneumonia, spontaneous pneumothorax.
- *Oesophageal reflux.* Hiatus hernia.

Pitfalls

- In herpes zoster, quite severe pain may precede the rash by some days.
- Ischaemic cardiac pain is often described as 'indigestion'. If 'indigestion' is severe enough to wake the patient up or to persist all night it is much more likely to represent angina or myocardial infarction.
- Ischaemic cardiac pain may be felt in the back, shoulders, arms, neck or face instead of, or as well as, in the central chest area.
- Left-sided inframammary pain is much more likely to be due to anxiety than angina.

Approach

History

Establish the site, onset, character and duration of pain, and ask about any associated symptoms – nausea, vomiting, faintness – and any precipitating and relieving factors.

Examination (essential to relieve anxiety)

Examine the cardiovascular system (CVS), respiratory system (RS) and BP.

Investigation

An *electrocardiograpm* (ECG) may be useful to demonstrate changes of infarction or arrhythmia, but remember a normal ECG at rest does not exclude angina or early infarction. It may help to reassure the patient. *Cardiac enzymes* should be repeated daily if infarction is suspected. *Chest x-ray* examination is indicated in smokers, immigrants, old patients, those with signs of pleurisy or pneumonia and persistent pain associated with cough.

Management

Determine patient's fears and reassure as appropriate, but if in doubt review the patient's condition within hours or days as required.

Severe chest pain demands powerful remedies, i.e. opiates by injection.

A decision about hospital admission must be made on clinical grounds.

COUGH

Most patients, or their parents, are more annoyed than worried by a cough. The temptation for a GP is to prescribe rather than try to make a diagnosis.

Common causes

- *Upper respiratory tract infection.* This is by far the most common cause of coughing, especially in children.
- *Bronchial irritation.* Smoking and, less commonly, dust and fumes are common causes of a persistent cough.
- *Asthma.* In many patients cough rather than wheeze is the predominant symptom, especially if it occurs on exercise or at night.
- *Chronic bronchitis.* The most common cause of a persistent, productive cough – especially if the patient is a smoker.

Less common causes

- *Pneumonia.*
- *Tuberculosis.* In immigrants, alcoholics and elderly men.
- *Carcinoma of bronchus.* In smokers, remember to have a chest x-ray if cough or physical signs persist after acute infection.
- *Foreign bodies* such as inhaled peanuts in toddlers.
- *Whooping cough.* In children, which is often modified by immunization.

Pitfalls

- Remember to think of allergy if the patient complains of frequent or persistent coughs and colds.

- Always consider the possibility of reversible airways obstruction, especially in children and elderly bronchitics.
- Remember that large numbers of eosinophils in sputum will colour it yellow, so allergy rather than infection may be the underlying cause of 'purulent' sputum.

Approach

History

Find out about smoking habits, and establish duration, severity and persistence of cough, and nature, consistency and colour of sputum. Find out if there is an association of chest pain or breathlessness.

Examination

Check general appearance, whether there is any weight loss or clubbing, and examine upper respiratory tract, including ears and chest.

Investigation

Chest x-ray examination in smokers, immigrants, older patients, pleurisy, pneumonia, whooping cough.

Peak-flow readings in asthma and bronchitis, before and after treatment.

Examine sputum for eosinophils. Cytology and culture may be useful occasionally.

Management

As appropriate, stop patient from smoking (and include parents). Remember that oral fluids and a humid atmosphere help expectoration and soothe cough, and most cough medicines are valueless but harmless.

Avoid giving antibiotics in uncomplicated upper respiratory tract infection (URTI).

Asthma requires bronchodilators and occasionally steroids, preferably by inhalation, rather than antibiotics.

INDIGESTION

Indigestion is a vague term used both by patients and GPs. It usually implies pain or discomfort felt in the epigastrium or lower chest. It may or may not be associated with heartburn, flatulence, nausea or vomiting.

Common causes

- *Dietary indiscretion.* Certain highly spiced foods (e.g. curry), salads, new bread or tomatoes, may cause indigestion in susceptible people.
- *Alcohol* is a common cause of recurrent indigestion.
- *Smoking.*
- *Excessive tea, coffee or mineral water.*
- *Drugs* especially aspirin.
- *'Stress', anxiety, depression.*

Less common causes

- *Peptic ulcer* typically causes recurrent bouts of dyspepsia over a 5 to 10 year period.
- *Hiatus hernia* is often symptomless, but may give rise to dyspepsia if there is acid reflux into oesophagus.
- *Gallbladder disease* is frequently symptomless, but may cause dyspepsia, jaundice and severe biliary colic.
- *Pancreatitis* is more common in alcoholics and diabetics.
- *Carcinoma of oesophagus, stomach* or *pancreas* are usually associated with dysphagia, anorexia, weight loss and malaise.

Pitfalls

- Avoid confusion with angina.
- Remember how common is alcohol abuse.
- Beware of the older patient who develops dyspepsia for the first time in his life – he may well have a malignancy.
- Remember to inquire about drug intake, especially self-medication.

Approach

History

Establish location and radiation of pain, aggravating and relieving factors, relationship to meals.

Find out response to self-medication – milk, antacids—and establish whether there are associated symptoms, especially melaena.

Examination

Check upper respiratory tract (URT) tongue, cervical lymph nodes, and examine abdomen – often nil specific to find.

Investigation

A *barium meal* may be indicated if symptoms persist or malignancy is a possibility. *Gastroscopy* may be a preferable initial investigation, depending on local conditions. *Ultrasound* is the quickest and cheapest way to demonstrate gallstones.

If *melaena* is suspected check occult blood in faeces. If *anaemia* is suspected check haemoglobin count.

Management

Tell the patient to avoid smoking, drinking, drugs and specific foods.

Suggest regular small meals and frequent and liberal doses of antacid.

The patient should avoid stooping, corsets, or horizontal position if reflux oesophagitis.

Give no specific ulcer treatment, e.g. cimetidine, without radiological or endoscopic proof.

Advise patient that most cases of nonspecific dyspepsia settle within a few days.

Acute

The GP must make a decision, not necessarily a diagnosis. Any signs of peritoneal irritation or obstruction indicate hospital admission even if the diagnosis is obscure.

Advise the patient to avoid food, emetics or purgatives.

Non-acute

Detailed history and careful examination is essential, but often the only treatment necessary is advice, especially dietary.

Investigations are indicated if the pain is persistent, unusual in that particular patient or associated with changes in bowel habit, bleeding or abdominal masses.

ABDOMINAL PAIN

Patients with abdominal pain are most likely to be worried about appendicitis or 'ulcers'. Older patients may have anxieties about cancer – they may be right.

Common causes

- In *young children. Colic* may cause severe spasmodic pain, often related to feeding problems or infection.
- In *older children.* Children may be 'little belly-achers', have the *periodic syndrome*—possibly equivalent to migraine – with recurrent central abdominal pain with or without vomiting.
- In *young adults. Indigestion* may be caused by stress, alcohol, nicotine, caffeine or irregular, unsuitable meals. Other common causes include irritable bowel syndrome, constipation and dysmenorrhoea.
- In *elderly patients. Constipation* or *diverticulitis* may be causes.

Less common causes

- In *young children. Urinary tract infection* or *intussusception* may be responsible.
- In *adults.* Patients may have *gallbladder colic, renal colic, peptic ulcer, colitis, Crohn's disease.*
- In *young women. Ectopic pregnancy, salpingitis* or *ovarian cysts* may be causes.
- In *the elderly.* An old person may have *acute* or *subacute obstruction* or *ischaemic bowel.*
- *All ages. Appendicitis* may be responsible.

Pitfalls

- Remember that as a GP you often see illness in its early stages. A careful examination may disclose nothing but a few hours later signs may be present. Be prepared to review the case if pain is persistent.

- Intussusception is often subacute rather than acute and may present in the same way as gastroenteritis.
- Appendicitis often presents atypically. It may follow gastroenteritis. Diagnosis is particularly difficult in children, pregnant women and the elderly.
- Remember extraneous causes, e.g. diabetic crisis, shingles.

BREAST LUMPS AND TENDERNESS

A lump in the breast inevitably raises fears of cancer in most women. To allay anxiety it is important for a GP to make a positive statement about his/her findings and proposed management.

Common causes

- *Normal cyclical changes* (worse if premenstrual). There is a wide range of variation between women, and between cycles in the same woman.
- *Mammary dysplasia* (cystic mastitis, fibroadenosis) may give rise to tenderness, thickening and cyst formation, age 25 to 50 years.

Less common causes

- *Fibroadenoma.* A firm, painless, mobile mass occurring predominantly in women under 30.
- *Carcinoma.* The hallmark is attachment to the skin or underlying tissues.
- *Breast abscess* is usually in the lactating breast.
- *Physiological mastitis* (neonate, puberty).

Pitfalls

- Carcinoma may occur in a woman with pre-existing mammary dysplasia.

Approach

History

Taking a family history is important, especially mother and sisters. Check her parity and lactation, and establish variability with cycle.

Examination

Both breasts and axillae should be examined, and establish shape, size, texture (whether soft, hard, cystic, or irregular) of lump if present. Find areas of tenderness. Look for axillary nodes.

Investigation

Arrange for a *mammography* if there are no definite physical signs, and in patients with previous breast cancer, strong family history, breast pain or very large breasts. It is most reliable in postmenopausal women.

Management

All isolated, persistent breast lumps must be regarded as malignant until proved otherwise. If mastitis is probable, review postmenstrually, but if sure there is no malignancy, reassure the patient strongly. If in doubt, refer the patient to a specialist.

DYSURIA AND FREQUENCY

Dysuria and frequency are most common in young adult women but are of most significance in children and adult men.

Common causes

- '*Cystitis*' which may or may not be associated with significant bacteriuria.
- *Urethritis.* Nonspecific urethritis (NSU) or gonorrhoea in men.

Less common causes

- *Pyelonephritis.* Fever and loin pain are typical features, more frequent in pregnancy, diabetics or in association with calculi.
- *Tuberculosis of genitourinary tract* in immigrants.
- *Bladder malignancy*, which is often associated with haematuria.
- *Prostatomegaly, prostatitis, carcinoma of prostate.*
- *Epididymo-orchitis.*

Pitfalls

- Urinary symptoms may be present in lieu of an underlying sexual problem.
- Urinary tract infection can occur without localizing symptoms, especially in small children.
- Prolapse in older women and prostatic problems in older men are often responsible for recurrent infections.
- Hormone deficiency in perimenopausal and postmenopausal women may cause recurrent urethral symptoms.

Approach

History

Establish whether there have been previous attacks, and find out if there are associated features. Ask about precipitating and relieving factors. Find out sexual and contraceptive habits.

Examination

Examine abdomen and loins for tenderness. Pelvic examination if indicated. Rectal examination in men.

Investigations

Mid-stream urine specimen (MSU) for culture and microscopy before prescribing antibiotics for children, adult men and pregnant women.

Intravenous urogram (IVU) or ultrasonic scanning may be required after treatment in children, adult men, women with recurrent infections or if calculi are suspected.

Management

Copious fluids by mouth or analgesics may be necessary. Antibiotics, e.g. trimethoprim or amoxycillin, should be prescribed if symptoms are severe.

Children and adult males should be referred to a specialist for further investigation. Recurrent 'cystitis' in adult women may require exclusion of precipitating factors and administration of prophylactic antibacterial drugs after intercourse, or at night.

PAIN IN THE BACK

Backache is common and disabling. The causes are legion and often unclear and most cases recover spontaneously. Nevertheless, it is a condition of great economic importance to the individual, to industry and to the state.

Common causes

- *Muscle* and *ligamentous injury* is usually associated with lifting, twisting and sudden movement.
- *Postural backache* is due to prolonged standing or sitting in unsuitable positions and is common in drivers and typists.

Less common causes

- *Prolapsed intervertebral disc* (PID) with low back pain and sciatica.
- *Bone pain* secondary to osteoporosis, malignancy or infection.
- *Osteoarthritis* in the elderly or after trauma.
- *Chronic depressive illness.*
- *Malingering.*

Pitfalls

- In PID, sciatica may occur without lumbago.
- Low back pain occurring for the first time after 50 years of age should be regarded with suspicion.
- Renal lesions or intra-abdominal conditions may produce referred pain in the back.
- Retention of urine in association with PID implies a central prolapse and demands urgent surgical intervention.

Approach

History

Establish the site, mode of onset, severity, radiation and duration of pain. Find out the precipitating and relieving factors and associated symptoms, e.g. urinary, abdominal.

Examination

Watch gait, mobility of spine, climbing on couch, and establish if there is local tenderness.

Examine on straight leg-raising and femoral stretch and establish tone, power, sensation and reflexes.

Examine abdomen, general condition and pulse rate (PR) if indicated.

Investigation

Nil in acute cases.

If persistent take *full blood count* (FBC), erythrocyte sedimentation rate (ESR), *biochemical profile* (including serum acid phosphatase), *serum electrophoresis, urinalysis*.

X-ray examination of lumbar spine, with or without chest, after severe pain has settled (no urgency required).

Management

Insist on strict rest on a firm surface, e.g. bed or floor, and give analgesics and local heat. Possibly give muscle relaxants. Laxatives are often required.

Most 'acute backs' will settle within 3 to 4 weeks on proper rest. Physiotherapy has a place in the rehabilitation phase of the 'acute back' and in the 'chronic back'. Manipulation may be helpful in the absence of positive neurological signs.

A few patients will require hospital admission for proper rest, epidural injection or surgery.

Subsequent attention to obesity, posture, working and living conditions is important if recurrence is to be avoided.

PAIN IN THE NECK

A 'pain in the neck' is used colloquially to describe someone or something which represents chronic irritation and annoyance.

Common causes

- *Acute torticollis.* Usually occurs in young adults during sleep.
- *Injury to muscles and ligaments*, e.g. whiplash in road traffic accident.

- *Cervical spondylosis.*
- *Osteoarthritis* or *subluxation of the apophyseal joints* in middle-aged and elderly people.

Less common causes

- *Prolapsed intervertebral disc* (usually C6-C7).
- *Generalized conditions*, e.g. rheumatoid arthritis, ankylosing spondylitis.
- *Bone pain* which is secondary to Paget's disease, malignancy and infection.

Pitfalls

- Remember to consider the neck as a source of pain presenting in the shoulder and arm.
- Because there is little space in the spinal canal at cervical level minor disc protrusions or tiny osteophytes can impinge on the cord or the vertebral arteries.
- Subluxation of the atlanto-axial joint in rheumatoid arthritis can lead to impingement of the odontoid process on to the cervical cord.

Approach

History

Establish site, mode of onset, severity, radiation and duration of pain. Find out precipitating and relieving factors, and associated symptoms, e.g. sensory, motor, joint pains, vertebrobasilar insufficiency.

Examination

Examine neck, posture, mobility for local tenderness, and examine shoulders and arms. Do neurological and/or general examination if indicated.

Investigation

Nil in acute cases.

   If persistent, *FBC, ESR, biochemical profile, electrophoresis, urinalysis*.

X-ray examination of cervical spine (special views may be required, check with radiologist).

Management

Rest, preferably in a soft collar, and give analgesics and local heat. Physiotherapy, manipulation or traction may be helpful if available. Local steroid injections are employed by some doctors. Cervical myelopathy demands urgent referral.

Suspicion of neoplasm, infection, serious trauma or an unsatisfactory response to simple treatment requires referral.

Recurrence is common, especially in mechanical lesions of the lower cervical intervertebral joints. It is worth advising the patient accordingly and keeping a soft collar available.

VAGINAL DISCHARGE AND IRRITATION

Vaginal discharge is a common nuisance which causes a great deal of discomfort and anxiety to women in their reproductive years.

Common causes

- *Excessive physiological secretion* during pregnancy, ovulation, premenstrually, while on the pill, or caused by 'erosion'.
- *Monilia with pruritus and soreness*, often thick and white discharge.
- *Trichomonas* causing soreness and intertrigo, often frothy and yellowish discharge.
- *Nonspecific vaginitis* (NSV) often has unpleasant smell due to *Gardnerella vaginalis*.

Less common causes

- *Venereal disease.* Chlamydia (NSU), gonorrhoea, herpes genitalis.
- *Malignancy* usually with bloodstained discharge.
- *Opportunist infections* such as intrauterine contraceptive device (IUCD), postpartum or postgynaecological surgery, retained tampons or other foreign bodies.
- *Atrophic vaginitis* (oestrogen deficiency) in postmenopausal women.

Pitfalls

* It is very difficult to exclude venereal disease in a woman, especially if it is coexisting with a vaginal infection. If in doubt, refer to a medical genitourinary clinic.

Approach

History

Establish whether there is pruritus, smell, need for protective wear and ask about sexual, contraceptive and menstrual history. Establish whether there is pain or discomfort.

Examination

Abdominal and pelvic examination. Distinguish between vaginitis, cervicitis and vulvitis.

Investigation

Urinalysis for sugar.

Take *cervical* and *vaginal swabs* in transport medium. Take *charcoal swabs* from urethra, cervix and rectum if gonorrhoea is suspected. Take a *cervical smear* (opportunity for screening).

Management

Give advice about hygiene, avoiding scented soaps, nylon pants, tights, bath salts, deodorants, etc., and give specific treatment, e.g. metronidazole for trichomonas; antifungal agent for monilia; antibiotics for chlamydia and gonorrhoea; and local oestrogens for atrophic vaginitis.

Arrange referral for: resistant or recurrent discharge; suspicion of sexually transmitted disease; and suspicion of malignancy.

ABNORMAL VAGINAL BLEEDING

This term covers many conditions, including intermenstrual bleeding, postcoital bleeding, menorrhagia, polymenorrhoea and metropathia haemorrhagica. Some complications of early pregnancy are also included.

Common causes

- *Contraceptive pill* problems especially spotting and breakthrough bleeding.
- *Threatened abortion* with vaginal bleeding with or without lower abdominal pain.
- *Cervical erosion* or *polyp* which is the commonest cause of intermenstrual and postcoital bleeding.
- *Hormonal imbalance*, which may cause anything from amenorrhoea to metropathia.
- *Fibroids*, often asymptomatic, may cause menorrhagia.

Less common causes

- *Malignancy of cervix* or corpus uteri.
- *Abnormal pregnancy* – ectopic, hydatidiform mole.
- *Endometriosis* is often associated with dysmenorrhoea and dyspareunia.

Pitfalls

- It is most important to clarify the position regarding contraception and the possibility of pregnancy.
- It is easy to confuse a carcinoma of the uterus with dysfunctional uterine haemorrhage.
- Do not rely on a negative cervical smear if clinically suspicious of malignancy.

Approach

History

Establish nature, type and pattern of bleeding (menstrual chart may help), and ask about any associated features such as pain, tiredness, symptoms of pregnancy. Take sexual and contraceptive history.

Examination

Abdominal and pelvic examination for tenderness, masses, discharge and inspection of cervix.

Investigation

Take a *cervical smear*. Take *cervical* and *vaginal swabs* if indicated. *Pregnancy test* if indicated. Arrange *haemoglobin estimation*.

Management

Reassurance alone may be all that is required, but if not give specific treatment, e.g. change of contraceptive pill; cyclical hormone therapy; or rest for threatened abortion.

Arrange referral for: suspected malignancy; endometriosis; large or symptomatic fibroids; inevitable, incomplete abortion or ectopic pregnancy (urgent admission).

DYSPAREUNIA

Dyspareunia may be superficial or deep and due entirely to organic or psychological causes, but commonly both factors will be present.

Common causes

- *Vulvovaginitis* from any cause.
- *Trauma* at first intercourse or postepisiotomy.
- *Psychosexual problems* are often associated with vaginismus.

Less common causes

- *Pelvic inflammatory disease* including cervicitis.
- *Endometriosis*.
- *Malignancy*.

Pitfalls

- Failure to take an adequate history may lead to inappropriate referral and even unnecessary operation.
- It is usually wise to exclude organic causes even if there are obvious psychosexual problems present.

Approach

History

Establish menstrual and obstetric history. Take psychosexual and contraceptive history and find out about associated features.

Examination

During abdominal and pelvic examinations note response to examination and take opportunity to clarify history.

Investigations

Cervical and *vaginal swabs* should be taken if indicated. Take a *cervical smear* (opportunity for screening).

Management

Give advice about nature of problem, and give specific treatment where possible and psychosexual counselling if appropriate.

Arrange referral for pelvic inflammatory disease; endometriosis; and major sexual problems.

PALPITATIONS

Palpitations are distressing and often worrying to patients because in the lay mind they are inevitably associated with heart disease.

Common causes

* *Paroxysmal supraventricular tachycardia* (SVT) which usually occurs in healthy adults.
* *Anxiety state* – fear, hyperventilation.
* *Ventricular extrasystoles* (VE) often described as extra beats or missed beats.

Less common causes

* *Paroxysmal atrial fibrillation* (PAF): patients are usually over 50 years of age.
* *Thyrotoxicosis* must be excluded.

- *Other cardiac arrythmias* that are usually associated with heart disease.

Pitfalls

- It is important to act decisively and reassure the patient confidently if heart disease can be excluded.
- Conversely, it is important not to reassure the patient if the diagnosis is uncertain and further investigation is indicated.
- Atrial fibrillation may be the only evidence of thyrotoxicosis, especially in the elderly.

Approach

History

Establish the nature, duration and regularity of palpitations, and find out the relationship to possible trigger factors – exercise, meals, smoking, alcohol, tea, coffee, anxiety. Also find out about associated features such as dyspnoea, angina, faintness. See if there are features of thyrotoxicosis.

Examination

Check pulse rate and rhythm and blood pressure; VEs are abolished by exertion, but PAF is not.
   Check CVS and RS.

Investigation

ECG (during attack if possible). Take *thyroid function tests*, if indicated. Chest *x-ray examination*.

Management

Give advice about smoking, drinking, tea, coffee, etc. reassure strongly if indicated. Apply vagal stimulation (eyeball pressure or carotid massage) for SVT.
   Give betablockers for SVT, thyrotoxicosis and give specific treatment for cardiac failure, ischaemic heart disease and valvular heart disease.

Arrange referral for elucidation of arrhythmia, specific anti-arrhythmic medication, and cardioversion.

HYPERVENTILATION

This is a common reaction to pain or anxiety, but occasionally is a pointer to serious underlying disease.

Common causes

- *Anxiety.*
- *Response to pain*, which may cause paraesthesia and tetany.

Less common causes

- *Respiratory disease* such as emphysema, pneumonia, asthma.
- *Diabetic keto-acidosis.*
- *Aspirin overdose.*

Pitfalls

- Failure to consider underlying disease if hyperventilation persists.

Approach

History

Establish facts about onset, precipitating factors and associated features.

Examination

This should be general (for reassurance).

Investigation

Not usually required.

Management

A calm, relaxed manner will reassure the patient. Suggest rebreathing from paper or plastic pag, and manage as appropriate for any underlying condition.

INSOMNIA

The amount of sleep which people require varies enormously from person to person. If a person feels well and functions normally then the duration and quality of sleep is adequate for that person.

Common causes

- *Shiftwork.*
- *External factors* such as noise, snoring partner, uncomfortable bed.
- *Anxiety/tension* often with a long history of difficulty in falling asleep.
- *Hypnotic dependence* developing tolerance to sedatives.
- *Ageing.* Sleep patterns change in the elderly.
- *Pain and discomfort.*

Less common causes

- *Depression* is classically associated with early waking.

Pitfalls

- Do not prescribe hypnotics before exploring underlying causes.
- Beware of attempted suicide by using an overdose of hypnotics.
- There is a danger of missing a depressive illness with serious results.

Approach

History

Ask about the pattern of sleep disturbance and previous sleep problems. Establish past psychiatric history, and find out if there are any social and emotional problems. Also find out about physical problems.

Examination

Examine if necessary to exclude physical disease.

Investigation

Usually unnecessary.

Management

Explain and reassure and give counselling if appropriate. Also give advice about relaxation and promotion of natural sleep, e.g. hot bath, hot drink, reading.

Suggest altering environment where possible, and give specific treatment for pain with analgesics; depression with antidepressants.

Hypnotics should be prescribed in small quantities for short periods only and barbiturates avoided.

Chapter 18

Planned professional services

As the doctor of first contact, the GP sees a number of patients who are not ill but who have consulted either for planned or preventive care, e.g. family planning, antenatal care, immunizations, or for certificates of one sort or another which only a doctor can provide.

Obviously if the practice provides a high-quality service in health education and preventive medicine it is of great benefit to both patients and doctors. Less obviously of benefit to the doctor is the provision of administrative services to his/her patients, but a helpful and considerate attitude by the doctor can strengthen his/her relationship with the patient thus helping it to withstand future strains more easily.

In this chapter we try to cover the main areas where patients consult not for illness per se, but for advice or for preventive or administrative action.

CONTRACEPTION

Most patients who come for contraceptive advice are either well established on a method or have clear ideas about which method they want to use.

If general advice is wanted or if the doctor does not think the method they are using or wish to use is likely to be safest or most reliable for them then remember the following:

- Discuss the advantages and disadvantages of all the feasible methods.
- The acceptability of the method to the couple may be as important as any medical consideration.

Method safety studies show that:

- Vasectomy is the safest and most effective method of contraception at any age.
- Female sterilization is better than any reversible method used for the same number of years.

- A barrier method combined with early abortion if unplanned pregnancy occurs is safe and effective.
- Deaths from the pill increase after the age of 35.
- Any method is safer than none.

Effective long-term use depends to a large degree on patient confidence and satisfaction with the standard of care they are receiving. Good care includes the following:

- An up-to-date well-informed GP who can fit both diaphragms and coils.
- An integrated screening programme so that rubella status is checked in nullips; 5-yearly smears are performed on all patients; and all patients are offered a leaflet or advice on self-examination of the breasts.
- A special contraceptive record card is kept in the notes.
- An intrapractice family planning clinic either run by the doctor or a family planning-trained practice nurse who can carry out pill, coil and diaphragm checks as well as fitting diaphragms and taking smears.

Fees may be claimed annually on forms FP 1001 or FP 1002 (see the Red Book).

The combined pill

The combined pill is virtually 100 per cent effective and best used
- Below the age of 35.
- When a couple wish to be certain no pregnancy will occur.
- If a woman suffers from any condition which the pill will benefit or relieve.

All varieties have $50\,\mu g$ of oestrogen or less and for practical purposes the choice of oestrogen or progestogen in the pill is unimportant.

Up to 3 days after unprotected intercourse two Ovran or Eugynon 50 tablets taken stat and again in 12 hours may provide postcoital contraception.

Absolute contraindications

The combined pill should not be used when any of the following conditions are present:

- Over 35-year-old women who smoke.
- Intravascular thrombosis including any condition predisposing to thromboembolism.
- Heart diseases including septal defects, mitral stenosis.
- Impaired liver function/porphyria/gallstones.
- Possible sex hormone-dependent tumours.
- Undiagnosed abnormal vaginal bleeding.
- Pregnancy.
- Pre-existing neuro-ophthalmic disorders.
- Pituitary dysfunction.
- Any condition that deteriorated appreciably in pregnancy.
- Recent hydatidiform mole.

Relative contraindications

Over 35 or over 30 if a woman is a smoker or she has any other risk factor, e.g.:

- Moderate hypertension.
- Obesity.
- Diabetes.
- Migraine.
- Lactation.
- Depressive states.
- Epilepsy.
- Oligomenorrhoea.
- Otosclerosis .
- Liver disorder.
- Renal disease.

Note: In these cases the combined pill represents a lesser risk than pregnancy, should no other method be acceptable or sufficiently effective, though special supervision is required.

Possible adverse effects

Minor side effects (nausea, irritability, breast tenderness, etc.) are common and usually disappear within a few cycles. As with loss of libido and depression, headaches including migraine are as likely to be improved as worsened by the pill though if headaches are precipitated by the pill or migraine worsened then the pill should be stopped.

Rarer more serious risks to health include thromboembolism, circulatory diseases, hypertension and gallstones – their incidence can be decreased by preprescription screening of users and careful follow-up monitoring.

Adverse effects do not include the development of diabetes, neoplasms or infertility.

Incidence reduction

Reduction of incidence of menorrhagia, dysmenorrhoea, premenstrual tension, mid-cycle pain, endometriosis, iron deficiency, anaemia, benign breast disease, carcinoma ovary, acne (in most patients).

Starting the pill

Before prescribing the pill assess risk factors and exclude contraindications from the history.

Check BP, note weight, institute screening programme, consider performing vaginal examination (do not insist if patient appears at all reluctant).

Explain how the pill works and how to take it (a leaflet may be helpful).

Prescribe a low dose pill, e.g. Ovranette, Microgynon, and ask patient to return in three months.

Follow-up

After initial 3 months patient should be seen 6-monthly with BP checked at every visit.

Review any problems or worries about pill use.

If breakthrough bleeding is occurring the most likely remedy in the first instance is to increase the progestogen (to Ovran 30 or Eugynon 30).

If the pill is not suiting the woman change from one preparation to another; this does not appear to lead to any loss of protection.

If a patient wishes to delay a period then she should take packets without a break.

The progestogen only pill (mini-pill)

The mini-pill is effective and best used in over 35-year-olds who do not wish sterilization and breast-feeding mothers.

Absolute contraindications

A recent hydatidiform mole and a history of ectopic pregnancy.

Relative contraindications

Hypertension, history of thromboembolism and risk factors for ectopic pregnancy.

Side effects

Bleeding abnormalities and breast soreness, but serious adverse effects are rare. If pregnancy occurs while on this pill then it may be ectopic.

Starting and follow-up.

As for the combined pill.

The intrauterine contraceptive device (IUCD) or coil

The IUCD is effective and best used as an alternative to the pill for those women who have at least one child; as an alternative to sterilization for women coming off the pill; and for the forgetful.

Absolute contraindications

- Pregnancy.
- History of ectopic pregnancy.
- Active pelvic inflammation.
- Undiagnosed irregular genital tract bleeding.

Relative contraindications

- History of pelvic infection.
- Nulliparity.
- Menorrhagia/anaemia.
- Previous caesarean section.
- Bleeding tendency/anticoagulation.
- Abnormalities of the uterine cavity.

Adverse effects

- If there is pregnancy it may be ectopic.
- Pelvic inflammation.
- Uterine bleeding and pain.
- Expulsion of the device.
- Perforation of the uterus.

Insertion techniques should be learned from training at a recognized centre. A GP who advises a patient to have a coil fitted, but does not fit coils, may refer the patient to a family planning clinic or hospital and claim the FP 1001 fee rather than the FP 1002. If pregnancy occurs with a coil *in situ* the patient should be referred to an obstetrician for removal of the coil.

Remove the coil by pulling threads with sponge forceps, downwards in direction of the long axis of the cervix. Best removed just after a period.

A coil inserted up to 7 days after unprotected intercourse will provide effective postcoital contraception because it interferes with implantation of the blastocyst.

Diaphragm and chemicals

The diaphragm is effective if used properly by a well-motivated woman. May be used in any age group by women who cannot or do not wish to take the pill.

There are no adverse effects and it may give protection against cervical cancer.

Spermicide must always be used and although the diaphragm may be fitted at any time before intercourse (extra spermicide if more than 6 hours before) it should not be removed until 6 hours after.

Training in fitting should be given by the practice family planning nurse or doctor.

The sheath

The sheath is much underrated, being potentially an effective, cheap and easy to use method.

Primary reasons for failure include the following:

- When it is not used on every conceivable occasion.
- When there is penetration before the sheath is put on.

- Failure to unroll the sheath to entire length or to leave sufficient space at the tip to act as ejaculate reservoir.
- Failure to withdraw while penis is still erect.

Sterilization

In either partner sterilization is safer and more effective than using any reversible method for the same number of years, but it should not be entered into lightly. It must be emphasized to the couple that for all practical purposes the procedures are irreversible.

There must be a full measure of counselling about medical and social factors and their implications for the future.

If all else is equal vasectomy is preferable to female sterilization because it is easier to perform and safer.

ABORTION COUNSELLING

The large majority of patients who consult have already made up their minds and do not want counselling but referral to an appropriate agency.

When others seem to be speaking for the patient she should be interviewed by herself to find out her real views.

The doctor should gather all the relevant facts before deciding what course to take.

- Refer for NHS abortion.
  – the views of the consultant the patient sees will determine whether abortion is carried out or not.
  – if carried out it is free.
  – best done before 12–13 weeks' gestation but can be done up to 20 weeks or more with prostaglandins.
- Refer for private abortion.
  – abortion will almost certainly be carried out.
  – costs more than £100.
  – in most areas it is likely to be safer, both in terms of mortality and morbidity, than an NHS abortion.
- Advise the patient to seek a second opinion from another doctor.
  – the doctor is supposed to do this if he/she has an ethical objection to referring patients for abortion.
- Advise the patient to consider proceeding with the pregnancy and keeping the baby or having it adopted.

– this advice is most unlikely to be heeded unless the patient is already working towards this decision herself.

The doctor's personal beliefs concerning abortion will determine the outcome of the consultation rather than any considered interpretations of the Abortion Act.

Modern abortion techniques, carried out before 12–13 weeks' gestation, do not appreciably impair future fertility. Patients who are refused abortion and go to term are more likely to suffer severe psychological disturbance than those who have abortions.

PRECONCEPTION COUNSELLING

There is increasing demand for this type of counselling and it can be useful. At present, it is usually provided in the context of a normal consultation and only when specifically requested. It will not be used by the majority of patients, unless it is well publicized as a service offered by the practice.

Objectives

- To help a couple consider all the implications of pregnancy and parenthood: practical, emotional, economic, social.
- To ensure that a couple are as healthy as possible at the time of conception and provide optimum conditions for conceiving a normal fetus.
- To detect any disease or disability which may need treatment before pregnancy or special care during it.
- To check rubella antibodies.
- To identify those who need genetic counselling.
- To identify those who will need to be seen especially early in pregnancy.
- To provide advice which will be needed between conception and the first antenatal visit.

Practice organization

Preconception advice can be provided by a nurse, health visitor or doctor, by appointment or in a specially designated clinic. Leaflets may be useful but cannot replace discussion and an opportunity to express anxieties and dispel unfounded fears. Both partners should be seen together.

What to include

Every couple

- General discussion about feelings and fears:
  – do they both want a baby?
  – is the relationship sound?
- Smoking: both partners should be non-smokers before conception.
- Alcohol: women should avoid alcohol around the time of conception, from the last period onwards, and keep it to a minimum thereafter.
- Oral contraception should be stopped and a barrier method used for at least one, preferably two or three, full cycles, before conception.
- Rubella antibodies should be checked.
- Healthy diet should be taken well before conception.
- Medicines: avoid over-the-counter medicines and make sure a patient her plans to any doctor who may prescribe for her.
- Medical checks: cervical smear, breast examination, BP and examination of the heart should have been done at some time during the year before conception. FBC will exclude anaemia.

Special groups

- A woman over 35 may wish to discuss her decreased likelihood of conception, risks of complications of pregnancy and delivery and of Down's syndrome.
- The implications of a previous abnormal baby or of a family history of inherited disorder will need to be discussed and possibly referred to a special centre for genetic counselling.
- Women with chronic diseases need special advice:
  – insulin-dependent diabetes: extra careful monitoring is needed from before conception. An insulin pump or frequent soluble insulin is usually advised before and during the pregnancy.
  – asthma: even short periods of hypoxia are disastrous to the fetus at any time. Control should be achieved before conception, using oral steroids, if necessary. They are well tolerated and less

likely to damage the fetus than hypoxia.
– congenital heart disease and hypertension should be assessed before conception as x-rays may be needed.
– long-term medication should be reviewed. Warfarin should not be taken during the first trimester.

• Patients at risk should discuss the possibility of aquired immuno-deficiency syndrome (AIDS) and consider having a blood test.
• Women in occupations which are hazardous in early pregnancy need special advice.

ANTENATAL CARE

In 80 per cent of cases, care is shared by a GP and specialist obstetrician. Unless there are problems, the bulk of the antenatal care is carried out by the GP with the hospital seeing the patient for booking, at 32 and/or 36 weeks, and at term.

In 20 per cent of cases care is provided solely by the GP, who also accepts the responsibility for backing up the midwife who supervises the delivery. Normally only those patients who, as far as one can predict, are going to have problem-free pregnancies and confinements are considered suitable for this type of care.

Objectives

• To prepare, educate, inform and help the expectant mother to achieve an enjoyable pregnancy, a safe delivery and a normal baby.
• To create and maintain good relations between the mother and the practice team (receptionist, health visitor, midwife and GP).
• To collaborate closely with local specialist obstetric and paediatric units.

Practice organization

This should ensure that:

• Antenatal care routines are clearly understood by patient and practice team.
• There are good shared records.
• There are speedy lines of communication with specialist services when difficulties arise.

- There are systems to keep late bookings to a minimum and to follow up defaulters and irregular attenders.
- There are clearly defined obstetric, medical and social risk factors which will lead to referral to specialist units.

An overall plan

Regular attendance is easier for patient and practice to follow, but flexibility may be necessary in individual cases. Present antenatal routines are outlined in Table 18.1.

Problems within this plan that should be considered include the following:

- Do all patients need iron and/or folic acid supplements and, if not, who does?
- What is the value of routinely listening to fetal hearts?
- Can antenatal care be humanized so that patients get time to talk about their worries rather than get processed mechanically?
- Why should patients be seen so often when likely pick-up rates for abnormalities, especially in the first 30 weeks, are so low? Would being seen at 8–12, 20, 26, 30, 34, 36 weeks and then weekly to term be as good?

Alphafetoprotein screening is now being carried out in many areas:

- Blood is best taken at 16–18 weeks (not before 16).
- Screening picks up 80–90 per cent of fetuses with open spina bifida and anencephalus.
- Couples must understand that a normal result does not guarantee a normal fetus.
- Only worth doing in patients who would consider termination should the result prove to be positive.

Amniocentesis should be offered to all pregnant women over the age of 36. It can pick up chromosomal abnormalities, e.g. Down's syndrome, open neural tube defects (fluid alphafetoprotein levels measured), and male fetuses at risk of a sex-linked disorder, i.e. if there is a risk of haemophilia it could show that the fetus was male but not whether that male would actually have haemophilia or not. There is the risk of spontaneous abortion in 1 per cent of cases, and it does not guarantee a normal fetus and should not be carried out unless termination would be considered should an abnormality be discovered.

Table 18.1 *Present antenatal routines for patient and practice*

Consultation	Practice staff or doctor	Doctor
Booking (8–12 weeks)	Fill in form FP24 of 24A Fill in personal details on cooperation card Weight Urinalysis (albumin/glucose) Blood pressure Fill in forms for: – Hb – ABO and Rhesus – Rubella antibodies – VDRL – MSU – Electrophoresis for abnormal Hb in women of African, Indian or Mediterranean extraction Take blood specimens	Full medical history Menstrual history Calculate expected date of delivery Past gynaecological history Past obstetric history Physical examination, including breasts, CVS, abdomen Anti-smoking propaganda Pro-breastfeeding propaganda Decide form and place of antenatal care and delivery Discuss patient worries/fears Fill in cooperation card
4-weekly (until 28 weeks)	Weight Blood pressure Urinalysis (albumin/glucose) Start iron/folic acid if indicated	Note when fetal movements felt Check fundus Discuss patient worries/fears
2-weekly (28–36 weeks) then weekly to term	Weight Blood pressure Urinalysis (albumin/glucose) Encourage care of breasts Arrange for parentcraft, relaxation classes, etc	Check fundus/fetal heart Confirm fetal position Check expected date of delivery Discuss patient worries/fears At 30 and 36 weeks check Hb, Rhesus antibodies if appropriate At 36 weeks check head engaged
Postnatal (6–8 weeks after delivery)	Weight Blood pressure Urinalysis (albumin/glucose) Send off completed form FP24 or 24A	Examine breasts and pelvis Cervical smear if indicated Discuss contraception Follow-up any antenatal or labour problems Complete form FP24 or 24A Complete form FP1001 or 1002 Inquire about baby's progress

CERVICAL CYTOLOGY

Smears detect dysplastic changes at the cervical squamocolumnar junction so allowing early treatment to prevent the development of invasive carcinoma.

In about 30 per cent of cases dysplasia, after an interval of 8–10 years, will progress to invasive carcinoma. Routine 5-yearly smears will therefore pick up the large majority of cases in time for effective treatment.

The first smear should be taken about age 20–25, usually after sexual activity has begun. Under certain circumstances a fee is claimable (see the Red Book).

To take a smear:

- Using a speculum, lubricated only with water, completely expose the cervix.
- With wooden spatula take a firm scrape of the squamo columnar junction through a full 360 degrees.
- Spread the material obtained thinly, to form a monocellular layer, on a glass slide.
- Fix the slide material with a solution of 95 per cent alcohol.

A practice screening policy (on whom, when, how often, by whom?) helps all partners and staff to give consistent advice. If a patient requests smears more often than seems appropriate then her reasons should be explored and advice given.

A well-trained practice nurse can run an intrapractice smear clinic with cases either self-referred, referred by the dotors or selected from the age–sex register.

If a smear is abnormal then the report will usually contain suggestions for appropriate action:

- Mild cases require repeat smears in 6–12 months.
- Severer cases or persistent mild cases require gynaecological referral for colposcopy.
- Trichomonas or thrush infection noted on a smear probably does not require treatment unless the patient has symptoms.

ASSESSMENT OF A CHILD'S DEVELOPMENT

Intensive developmental screening is of unproved value. Doctors who hold regular intrapractice developmental clinics argue that giving support and advice to parents is as important as the detection of abnormalities.

Whether a formal practice screening policy exists or not every GP should, at any consultation concerning a child, be looking for and recognizing defects outside the range of normal. A GP should also be able to make a reliable appraisal of a child's development and give sound guidance in answer to parents' questions.

Development

A child's development is of increasing complexity while growth is increasing. It takes place in various different ways (locomotion, manipulation, use of eyes and ears, speech, etc.) and though all babies follow the same sequence of development the rate varies from child to child. Even the same child does not develop at a constant rate but in lulls and spurts.

Uniformly retarded development implies mental retardation or severe emotional deprivation. Slowness in one particular field is not a sign of retardation but may be due to a family trait; lack of stimulation; or physical disease.

Progress depends on the maturing of the central nervous system and so cannot be accelerated by outside stimulation. On the other hand, illness and environmental factors may retard it.

Assessment

This requires answers to the following questions:

- Is this child developing normally?
- Is the child's behaviour appropriate for its age?
- Does the child still exhibit signs of earlier behaviour which by now should have gone?
- Are there any abnormal signs?

Infants with major abnormalities and abnormalities which might have important consequences should be referred to a (developmental) paediatrician. So should any infant which has not reached an important milestone at the age when most infants would have been expected to. The age when most infants should possess an ability is known as the limit age. Some important limit ages are shown in Table 18.2.

DISCUSSION OF WHOOPING COUGH VACCINATION

Since concern over the safety of pertussis vaccination was first voiced in 1974 the percentage of children under 2 who are vaccinated has

Table 18.2 *Developmental delay at various age limits*

Referral age	Behaviour
6 months	Head still wobbly Fists clenched Not reaching with hands
12 months	Not able to sit without support Not able to take weight on legs Not transferring between hands Not looking Not listening
18 months	Not walking alone Not vocalizing Still casting objects Still mouthing
24 months	Not saying a single word Not showing any imagination or imitation in play Lack of interest

dropped from 78 to 38 per cent and there has been a major rise in the incidence of whooping cough (102,000 cases notified in the 1977–9 epidemic). The panic is now over and the percentage of children immunized is over 60 per cent.

Parents may seek advice before having their baby vaccinated. Some points are worth making:

- Whooping cough is a serious disease that can cause death as well as an unknown number of cases of brain and lung damage.
- Of children below the age of 2 with whooping cough, 10 per cent have to be admitted to hospital.
- Medical treatment is unsatisfactory.
- Vaccination is over 90 per cent effective.
- Minor reactions to vaccination (irritability, pyrexia, sore arm, vomiting) occur in up to 10 per cent of cases and resolve within 24 to 48 hours.
- In children who are potential febrile-fitters a vaccine-induced fever may provoke a fit but fits are common at this age anyway and there is no evidence that the vaccine causes fits directly.
- The vaccine does cause some cases of serious brain damage. If all 600,000 children born in Britain each year undergo a full course of pertussis vaccination then six will have a severe reaction and be left with a permanent disability (75 per cent of the children

developing serious reactions will do so within 24 hours of vaccination).

Contraindications to vaccination

- Where there is a history of fits in the child or close family history of fits (parents, sibs, grandparents).
- Where there is any abnormality of the central nervous system.
- Where there has been a severe reaction to a previous dose of triple vaccine (no more pertussis, but continue with the others).
- When the child has an acute illness with a fever (wait until better and then vaccinate).

For normal children, without contraindications, the benefits of vaccination outweigh the risks, though only the parents can decide what is best for their child. If the doctor's own children have been vaccinated, telling the parents so will be more useful than making any number of medical points.

It is vital that the entire practice (partners, health visitors, nurses) follow the same guidelines for advising parents. Team members may well benefit from intrapractice teaching or discussion on this topic.

IMMUNIZATION FOR A CHILD

In many practices routine immunizations are carried out by the practice nurse and not the doctor. The doctor remains responsible for the nurse's actions and must ensure that she is fully trained and competent. Regular teaching sessions are necessary.

Schedule

- Diphtheria/tetanus/pertussis (triple) and polio immunization at 3, $4\frac{1}{2}$, $8\frac{1}{2}$–11 months.
- MMR (measles, mumps, rubella) at 15 months.
- Diphtheria/tetanus and polio immunization at $4\frac{1}{2}$ years.
- If pertussis not wanted or contraindicated then give diphtheria/tetanus immunization.
- In the event of a whooping cough outbreak a crash regimen of three doses of triple at monthly intervals from the age of 3 months may be given. A diphtheria/tetanus booster than has to be given at 12–18 months.

Table 18.3 *Administration of vaccine for immunization of child*

Vaccine	Dose	Adverse effects	Notes
Triple	0.5 ml. × 3 i.m. or deep s.c.	Transient local erythema and tenderness Restlessness and irritability in 24 hours after vaccination Occasional screaming fits Rarely encephalopathy	If only first dose given then two doses at about six months' interval needed If only first two doses given then third will probably be effective up to 12 months after the second
Polio (Sabin)	3 drops × 3 oral	Rarely vaccine related paralysis in recipients or contacts	Unvaccinated parents of a child being immunized should also be offered immunization
MMR	0.5 ml i.m. or deep s.c.	Usually about 8th day with mild cough, cold, rash, occasionally mild parotitis pyrexia Rarely high pyrexia and febrile fit Encephalitis in 1 in 1 million cases	Children with a personal or close family history of fits should be given MMR provided parents understand that there may be a febrile response.

Contraindications

- *Diphtheria.* No contraindications but should not be given to people over the age of 10 years unless they are Schick-positive.
- *Tetanus.* None, but once the basic course is complete there should be at least one year between boosters.
- *Pertussis.* See page 116. Additionally should not be given to any child over the age of 3 years.
- *Polio.* Immunological dysfunction; malignant disease; steroid therapy; immunosuppressant therapy; radiotherapy; past history of adverse reaction to penicillin; within 3 weeks of another live vaccine; pregnancy (in adults). If diarrhoea and vomiting or an acute febrile illness are present vaccination should be postponed.
- *MMR.* As for polio but also including active tuberculosis; allergy to egg.

Administration

See Table 18.3.

Waiting for babies to be brought for immunizations is not enough. Use of the age–sex register, or a card index system, allows a record to be kept of each baby vaccinated – those who are shown to have missed vaccinations can then be actively followed up by the health visitor.

A LETTER OR CERTIFICATE FOR A THIRD PARTY

GPs have access to considerable amounts of information about their patients. They are also considered to be unbiased and truthful in a way that individual patients are not.

A great variety of bodies (employers, DHSS, councils, social services, lawyers and insurance companies) will approach GPs for verification of information that a patient has already given them or for a medical opinion to help them assess a patient's capabilities or needs.

If the approach comes through the patient the following should be remembered:

- Implied consent is given for the release of confidential information.
- In many cases a fee may be asked for but, depending on individual circumstances, this is often waived.
- If a fee is payable by the official body, provided that they have approached the doctor directly, the patient should be advised to ask them to write.
- Even when a request seems frivolous or vexatious, before refusing out of hand remember that the patient may be trapped between two powerful bodies, *viz* the GP and the third party, and the GP is likely to be the more sympathetic. Giving the patients what they need and then writing strong letters to the bodies concerned may be the best line of action.

If the approach comes directly from a third party the following applies.

- The patient's explicit written authority for the release of confidential information is necessary.
- Even if there is written authority, should it seem possible that the patient does not appreciate the implications of what is going to be disclosed he/she should be interviewed first.
- Keep a record of the fee owed so that a payment reminder may be sent if the bill is not met in good time.

A MEDICAL CHECKUP

It is transparently obvious to the layperson that a checkup is a good thing to have and so checkups are gaining in popularity. Problems posed in practice are as follows:

- Checkups are time-consuming procedures.
- There is no objective evidence that they are of any real benefit.
- There is no extra fee for service under the NHS, and no private fee is allowable.
- There is no agreed standard programme.
- There are no special NHS records for the exercise.

A request for a checkup may be a cry for much more than a physical examination and personal and family psychosocial matters should be explored.

While the GP would be within his/her rights to refuse to perform a checkup perhaps the opportunity could at least be used to discuss personal health risk habits and to check the blood pressure.

OVERSEAS TRAVEL ADVICE

Prospective travellers will consult primarily for vaccinations, but some may come to ask for prescriptions for travel sickness pills, antidiarrhoeal mixtures or even calamine lotion. Do not prescribe, but advise that such medicines may be bought from the chemist.

The DHSS booklet *Notice to Travellers – Health Protection* may be obtained free from the DHSS and given to each overseas traveller.

General advice

- Never trust the cleanliness of drinking water unless you are sure it has been boiled and never drink milk that has not been pasteurized or boiled.
- Bottled or aerated waters should be safe to drink.
- Do not eat unwashed vegetables or fruit unless they have an intact detachable cover, e.g. oranges.
- Check safety of all swimming areas before bathing.
- Take out adequate medical insurance cover.
- If ill for any length of time seek reliable medical advice (bank, embassy, airline will give you a safe contact).
- Take a small medical kit containing paracetamol, codeine phos-

Table 18.4 *Vaccinations needed in various parts of the world (view with Table 18.5)*

Area	Vaccinations (* mandatory)
South Europe	Polio
Central and South America	Yellow fever*, typhoid, polio
Middle East	Typhoid, cholera, polio
North Africa	Typhoid, cholera, polio
Central, East and West Africa	Yellow fever*, typhoid, polio
South Africa	Typhoid, polio
Indian subcontinent	Typhoid, polio
South-East Asia and China	Typhoid, polio

phate (for diarrhoea), antifungal powder, antiseptic cream, band-aid plasters, antimalarials.

Immunization

Many travellers do not consult early enough to allow for optimal spacing of vaccinations – a rapid scheme may be used though less effective immunity is gained.

Travellers to northern Europe, North America, Japan, Australia and New Zealand require no particular immunization though tetanus booster may be indicated, especially for campers. For other areas of the world check Table 18.4 then Table 18.5 to plan individual programme.

See the Red Book for fees that are claimable from the NHS for overseas vaccination. If no fee is claimable or if an international certificate is required you may charge a private fee (see BMA booklet; establish practice policy).

- For all countries check if tetanus toxoid needed, especially by campers or overland travellers.
- For overland travellers and those going to primitive regions use human normal immunoglobulin (HNIG) for prophylaxis against hepatitis A.
- For travellers (not holidaymakers) to primitive regions give rabies vaccine.
- Smallpox vaccination should not be required by any traveller.

Malaria prophylaxis

It is not possible to guarantee prevention.

Table 18.5 *Vaccine programme*

Yellow fever (live)	Given at special centres One injection gives immunity for 10 years Not within 2 weeks of polio or gammaglobulin
Typhoid (killed)	Two doses at 4–6 week interval 3-yearly boosters if still exposed to risk
Cholera (killed)	Two doses at 1–4 weeks' interval 6-monthly booster if still exposed to risk International certificate of vaccination required for entry into some countries
Polio (live)	Three doses at six weeks then 6-month intervals 5-yearly booster Not within 2 weeks of yellow fever or gammaglobulin
Tetanus (toxoid)	Three doses at four weeks then 6-month intervals 10-yearly booster
Gammaglobulin	Protects against hepatitis A for up to 6 months Give 4 days or so before travel

Note: For all vaccinations look up dosage, route of administration, contraindications and side effects on the label or notes accompanying the vaccine.

General measures

- Wear long sleeves and trousers, especially during evenings.
- Use insect repellant.
- Sleep under a mosquito net.

Drugs

- Drugs are needed for even a one day stay in a malarial area.
- Tablets should be taken at least 1 week before travel and continued until 6 weeks after return to the UK.
- Recommended regimens change according to the appearance of resistant strains and advice should be sought from the nearest centre.
- The choice of drugs is between the following:
    - paludrine 200 mg daily with chloroquine 300 mg weekly.
    - chloroquine 300 mg weekly with maloprim 1 tablet weekly.
    - paludrine 200 mg daily.
    - paludrine 100 mg daily.
- Children and pregnant women need special regimens.

REFERRAL FOR A SECOND OPINION (see also pages 52-4)

In any year up to 20 per cent of persons in the UK are referred by GPs to consultants for their specialist opinion and technical expertise. On average, a GP will write eight referral letters a week and the best ones will be brief and to the point explaining what the problem is, what investigations or treatment has been carried out, why referral is taking place and what is expected from the consultant.

A cardinal ethical rule is that no consultant should see a patient without a GP's referral letter. This still holds true for NHS patients, though many consultants are happy to give their opinion to unreferred patients prepared to pay for the privilege.

In many cases where the GP has not thought of getting a second opinion a patient's request for referral may come as quite a surprise. The doctor may feel upset, hurt, bewildered, rejected or even angry.

The doctor's feelings notwithstanding, the patient's wishes should be calmly explored.

- Is the patient unhappy with the doctor's care? If so, in what way?
- Does the patient not believe or not accept the diagnosis (or lack of it)?
- Are the implications of the diagnosis such that a different opinion is desired?
- Does the patient, or relatives, feel that alternative or better treatment is available elsewhere?

Discussion may result in the following.

- The patient's fears or worries being allayed so that the relationship with the doctor is strengthened.
- An improvement in the standard of care or, at the least, the patient's perception of it.
- A reasonable referral instituted, without acrimony, either through the NHS or privately.
- A totally unreasonable request turned down after obviously careful consideration and explanation.
- A recognition that the doctor–patient relationship has totally broken down and that it would be best for the patient to see a different doctor.

For patients who have a habit of constantly seeking second opinions, without paying much attention to the first, the GP must decide whether he/she can live with this behaviour or whether the patient should be asked to leave his/her list.

AIDS

The impact of the AIDS epidemic has stimulated plans and actions on prevention, relief and comfort, since there is no cure yet.

Public health education has been extensive and intensive and everyone must know about AIDS and its general implication.

There are special roles for the GP in personal care. Vulnerable individuals should be defined during routine consultations. Those particularly at risk are homosexual and bisexual men, injecting drug users, haemophiliacs, the sexual partners of these individuals and those who have had sexual contacts in parts of Africa. These groups of people should be counselled on prevention by reducing the number of sexual partners, knowing about a partner's previous sexual and drug history and by using a condom.

Although the prevalence of AIDS and HIV infection is likely to be very low in most practices the GP is likely to be asked for blood tests by anxious individuals and a policy should be developed in consultation with the local pathology laboratory. The GP should also be prepared to advise possible at-risk persons to have screening tests for HIV antibodies.

Each district has plans for treating persons with AIDS and care has to be carefully coordinated.

TERMINAL CARE

It is likely that a GP with 2000 patients may be involved in home care for about three terminally ill persons each year. This will involve close collaboration with the district nurses and the hospital services and perhaps with a local hospice, if there is one.

Every GP should be able to provide good terminal care involving personal support for the family as well as the patient and he/she should develop a programme for relief of pain and other common symptoms of the dying.

Chapter 19

Emergencies

RESPONSIBILITIES

A GP is obliged by the terms of service to provide 24-hour medical care for patients. He/she must also respond to emergency calls for any patients in the practice area if the patient's own doctor is not available.

A GP is *not obliged* to visit on request – only as the occasion demands. Responsibility for the decision is the doctor's.

If the duty is delegated to a doctor who is *not* on the Family Practitioner Committee (FPC) list, the delegating doctor retains responsibility for the deputy's actions.

Practice staff should be able to apply basic first aid, resuscitation and life support measures.

Preparation and equipment

The visiting bag

The exact contents are an individual matter though your trainer is likely to have fairly firm ideas about what you should be carrying.

Equipment in the car

- Nebulizer or Nebuhaler.
- Brook airway.
- Spare syringes, path bottles.
- Oxygen-giving set.
- Saline drip set.
- Torch and map of the area.
- List of telephone numbers – hospitals, ambulance, etc.
- Supply of forms, letter paper, etc., in car or bag.

Note: Make sure that the car is reliable.

The house

Have a telephone extension in your bedroom. Get your line listed as an emergency number. This gives you priority for repairs.

Ideally you need someone in the house to answer the telephone when you are out on a call. If you live alone you will need an answering machine.

Familiarize yourself with telephone procedures.

Telephone answering

Virtually all emergency calls are made by telephone. A kind considerate manner will enable you to get information while keeping the caller happy.

You are not obliged to visit, but if the caller is in a panic, or aggressive, *visit first*. Explain and educate later. If you are going to visit say so early on because this allays anxiety. Advice should be clear and simple.

Encourage the caller to ring back if the situation changes or if worried.

The most important item of information is the patient's *name and address*.

The nature of emergency calls

Several surveys show that most calls are not frivolous.

Young parents who have little knowledge of illness become acutely anxious about symptoms that appear trivial to the doctor. The call may reflect the fact that the family is under stress, or that the extra anxiety cannot be tolerated. It may be used as a weapon. Relatives who do not want to become involved in caring will often pass on responsibility by calling the doctor.

Anxiety in the caller may cause an aggressive manner. Previous contact with unwilling doctors may also cause aggression in an effort to ensure a visit.

Appropriate action

Direct patient to hospital if major trauma, burns or poisoning. Call ambulance. Only go yourself if you can do something useful.

Visit if medically indicated or if caller's anxieties and expectations are such that advice will not be tolerated when the problem is discussed on the telephone.

Give advice for simple illnesses where caller is satisfied and intelligent enough to understand instructions.

Principles of management in the home

- A calm methodical approach is vital even if you are cross or worried.
- A careful history and examination gets you the information you need as well as having a calming effect on the patient.
- Deciding on correct disposal is more important than making an accurate diagnosis.
- Give clear and simple instructions – written if necessary.
- Educate at every opportunity, but only after you have examined and made your decisions.
- Make careful notes.
- Arrange for any necessary follow-up.

ADMISSIONS

Reasons for admission

Where there is a medical necessity and/or social conditions make home care difficult.

When there is abuse of children or elderly, and when admission is demanded by patient or relative (rare).

Responsibility

Having made the decision that an admission is necessary, it is the GP's duty to implement this.

Contact local hospitals: if there is no bed, contact consultant. If no help there, contact medical referee of Hospital Bed Bureau (you can get the telephone number from the hospital or district health authority).

Arrange for an ambulance giving degree of urgency.

Send letter with full information including details of allergies and drug treatment. Be honest about reasons for admission.

CLINICAL MANAGEMENT

In this book it is not possible to give a complete guide to the management of all emergencies, but some problems which are either unique to general practice, or which present particular problems for the trainee, are as follows.

PAEDIATRIC EMERGENCIES

Special problems

- A great many out-of-hours calls are for acute illnesses in children.
- Parents, especially the young and isolated, are very anxious.
- Listen carefully to parents – they are often right about their child, even when you cannot find anything wrong.
- Repeated or unnecessary calls may be due to: excessive anxiety, family stress, child abuse, or low intelligence.
- The clinical condition of children changes rapidly, so always be willing to see the patient again to reassess.

The examination

- Patience and tolerance are needed.
- Small children are calmer if examined on the mother's lap.
- All systems must be examined every time. The symptoms of small children are not well localized, e.g. otitis media may be the cause of vomiting.
- Undress the child (take nappy off).

Child abuse

Always be on the lookout for evidence of mental or physical abuse. Abuse is often associated with:

- Low birth-weight babies.
- Babies who have been separated from mother soon after birth.
- Young parents.
- Social or emotional difficulties.
- Frequent attendances at surgery or casualty.
- Children with feeding problems, crying and vomiting.

Parents at the end of their tether may be anxious or aggressive.

Potential abuse

If you detect excessive tension ask the parents in a kind and sympathetic way if they sometimes feel violent. Offer maximum support from yourself, the health visitor, or from social services.

If the situation is tense then admit the child to hospital to allow the crisis to cool off.

Established abuse

Admit immediately to hospital, if abuse is established, and inform social services.

The crying child

A crying child is a frequent reason for an emergency call and generates much anxiety in parents and doctor.

Crying of acute onset

Severe crying or screaming in a normally happy child is significant.

Assessment

Find out if crying is associated with being touched or moved, or with defaecation or micturition. Does the child draw up legs? Is it episodic? Any recent trauma or illness? Examine carefully – particularly ears, abdomen, genitalia and bones, and test for meningism.

Common causes are:

- Otitis media.
- Abdominal pain – often colic (remember intussusception).
- Osteomyelitis.
- Fracture (remember abuse).
- Strangulated hernia.
- Torsion of testicle.
- Inflamed foreskin – pain on micturition.
- Inflamed perianal area due to diarrhoea.

Management

Treatment of the underlying condition. If no cause is found, the child may need admission for observation.

The always crying child

The emergency call is usually because parents have reached the end of their tether. They may be aggressive – 'There must be something wrong with him.'

Watch out for potential baby battering.

Assessment

Carefully examine child to reassure parents. Typically the baby is well and gaining weight.

Management

Reassurance and support from you or health visitor. If baby is at risk *admit*.

The feverish child

Other symptoms often indicate the cause of the fever but it is the fever itself that usually worries the parents.

Indications for a visit

- If the children are young – especially below 2 years of age.
- Where there is a very high temperature or history of febrile convulsions.
- When the child is excessively drowsy or irritable.
- When parents are very anxious.
- Where there is no obvious cause or possible serious cause for fever.

Telephone advice

- Reassure – fever is not in itself dangerous.
- Keep the child cool and give plenty of fluids.

- Use paracetamol only if the child is irritable.
- Call again if fever persists or if child gets worse.

Assessment and management

Do a careful examination of the child to find the cause and treat accordingly. If there is a clear risk of a febrile fit, give 0.25 mg/kg rectal, diazepam (Valium).

Do not use antibiotics unless there is a clear indication.

The child with croup

Croup is the symptom complex of an explosive cough, a hoarse voice and stridor. It is caused by acute laryngotracheobronchitis, acute epiglottitis or a foreign body.

Acute laryngotracheobronchitis

It may precede a cold, it is mildly febrile and not very toxic, and there is a pronounced cough with high-pitched stridor.

Acute epiglottitis

Onset is sudden and may be preceded by a sore throat. The child is very toxic, leaning forward and sitting still. Low-pitched stridor with little or no cough.

Foreign body

A foreign body may lead to a sudden onset of coughing and stridor with no fever.

Stridor

Assessment

Severe obstruction is indicated by:

- Marked stridor all the time.
- Child lies quiet and may be drowsy.
- The skin is pale and lips blue.

- There may be a distinct use of accessory muscles and intercostal recession.

Do not examine the throat if there is any suspicion of acute epiglottitis as this may precipitate respiratory and cardiac arrest.

Management

Admit if there is any suspicion of epiglottitis; moderate or severe croup; or suspicion of foreign body.

Keep at home if there is croup with mild stridor (treat with steam and amoxycillin); parents to stay up with the child; and call again if condition worsens.

The child with asthma

Any lower respiratory tract infection may be associated with wheezing. Recurrent wheezy bronchitis is usually asthma and should be treated with bronchodilators rather than antibiotics.

A visit is advisable if the parents are worried by the child's breathing.

Assessment

The amount of audible wheezing is a poor indication of the severity of the bronchospasm. In severe bronchospasm the child lies still, is anxious and does not talk, is pale with blue lips, and there is intercostal recession and use of accessory muscles. There is poor air entry – *beware* silent chest.

Management

One year and under (but is more likely due to bronchitis or bronchiolitis). Admit if bronchiolitis. If kept at home use steam, amoxycillin (if chest infection present).

Two years and over. Try two puffs Bricanyl inhaler using Nebuhaler. If the child is unable to use Nebuhaler then deliver aerosol to the face by using half the plastic bubble as a 'mask'.

If inhaler effective then leave inhaler and advise parents to give two puffs 3 hourly, whether child wheezy or not, until child seen again. If available use nebulizer.

If inhaler not effective and wheeze moderate or severe give subcutaneous terbutaline (Bricayl):

> 2 years 0.1 mg s.c.
> 5 years 0.2 mg s.c.
> 10 years 0.3 mg s.c.

If effective treat as inhaler effective above. If still not effective admit and give i.v. hydrocortisone 100 mg before transfer.

The recurrent wheezer

Parents should keep a stock of suitable drugs at home. If known to have severe or persistent attacks may be given prednisolone to use in short courses.

The child who has fits

One child in 12 will have had a seizure of some sort by the age of 11 years. These are most likely to be febrile fits but if recurrent may be epilepsy.

The caller is usually very upset and is often afraid that the child is dying.

The risk of structural cause or subsequent epilepsy is greatest if: fit is prolonged; fits start below age of one year; it is a focal fit; or there are recurrent fits.

Telephone

Tell caller you will visit immediately and to put child into the recovery position and, if febrile, start tepid sponging.

Management

If fit has stopped, take careful history to establish whether it was a fit.

- If first fit admit to hospital.
- In recurrent fits, if there is any suspicion that it may be meningitis – *admit*. Otherwise treat exactly as before, but keep at home; give tepid sponging; paracetamol; rectal diazepam (Valium) 0.25 mg/kg (use a syringe without a needle).

If still having fit, i.v. diazepam (Valium) 0.125 mg/kg slowly. If you cannot get into a vein give rectal diazepam (Valium) 0.25 mg/kg. Then admit.

Follow-up

If the child is kept at home revisit after two hours. If there are recurrent fits consider need for prophylactic treatment.

The child with vomiting or diarrhoea or both

Vomiting and diarrhoea in a child may be associated with almost any physical or emotional illness. This is particularly true of vomiting. The younger the child the less specific are the symptoms. The importance of these symptoms is related entirely to the underlying cause and the extent of any associated dehydration.

Telephone

Make sure of what the caller means. Posseting or the normal loose stools of a baby may be regarded with alarm by inexperienced parents. The younger the child and the iller the child, the more important it is to see the child.

Assessment

Make a careful examination and history to determine the cause. In particular, check for otitis media, tonsillitis, meningitis or any abdominal disaster. Look for signs of dehydration: dry mouth, dry nappy, slack skin, depressed fontanelle and drowsy apathetic behaviour.

Management

Treatment, if any, should be for underlying cause. If gastroenteritis no antibiotics. If severe take a faecal sample for culture. For fluid replacement, give little and often – hourly if possible. Use water or Diorylate (sodium chloride and dextrose oral powder compound), one sachet per 200 ml water, or lemonade or icecream soda for older children. *Do not* use salt or drinks with a lot of glucose.

Follow-up

Infants, if at all ill, must be revisited. Advise parents to call again if the child's condition deteriorates.

Abdominal pain in children

Most parents are worried about appendicitis when they call. This is likely to be uppermost in the doctor's mind as well. In virtually every instance the child must be seen, though if the history is short then a judicious delay may make diagnosis and assessment easier.

Assessment

Abdominal pain is often the presenting symptom of disease of other systems, so all systems need to be examined. Examine abdomen with great patience in the wriggling toddler, just keep your hand gently on the abdomen while the child is being cuddled on mother's lap.

Causes to remember

- *Evening colic* in babies under 3 months. It is recurrent, the baby is well, parents anxious.
- *Colic* due to gastroenteritis or respiratory tract infections.
- *Intussusception.* Commonest at age 5–9 months. Severe colic but well in between spasms. Look for blood and take pulse rate.
- *Strangulated hernia or torsion of testes.* Lower abdominal pain – diagnosis will be missed if child is not undressed.
- *Appendicitis.* Often atypical in children – hence the need for obsessionally careful abdominal examination. If in doubt always re-examine later. It is dangerous to make a diagnosis of mesenteric adenitis.
- *Urinary tract infections.* Urinary symptoms are often absent. High index of suspicion needed. Take mid-stream urine specimen.

Management

Treat underlying cause and admit if there is any suspicion of a surgical condition. Keep at home with clear instructions to call again if any worse. Revisit if any cause for anxiety.

EMERGENCIES IN ADULTS

Abdominal pain

Principles of management

Acute abdominal pain causes great anxiety in patients and relatives who always worry about appendicitis. Beware of bias, even in the most chronic of neurotics. They are just as likely to get an acute abdomen as anybody else.

Always see the patient – pain may sometimes be due to a severe disorder.

Assessment

A careful history will usually give you the diagnosis, but you will be caught out sooner or later if you do not perform a scrupulous examination including hernial orifices, bowel sounds and a rectal examination.

Appropriate disposal is more important than accurate diagnosis. The most important decision is: 'Is this an acute surgical condition?' Marked tenderness, guarding, rebound tenderness and constant pain all point to a surgical condition. Do not forget that in the early stages of obstruction the pain may be colicky with no physical signs in the abdomen.

Management

If acute surgical condition is suspected *admit*. If the condition is medical/cold surgical keep the patient under surveillance and try to reach a precise diagnosis. Refer as necessary.

Psychosocial emergencies

Such emergencies are not very common but incidence does vary with practice area. They are disproportionately difficult to deal with. Formal diagnosis is not as important as the degree of disturbance that the patient is causing. Aberrant behaviour may be understandable in terms of reaction to events in the patient's life and is not a sign of mental illness.

The mental state of other involved people may be relevant – who is really the patient?

Resist being blackmailed into accepting responsibility for a problem unless you are convinced that the patient is unable to make logical decisions. Do not label a patient as 'mad' if there is any reasonable doubt.

Symptoms

Confusion

The patient is disorientated in time and place, but usually has lucid intervals, and is often restless and panicky. Hallucinations are possible. Condition is generally worse at night.

In the young it may be due to drugs or alcohol.

In the elderly it may be caused by cerebral arteriosclerosis with underlying illness.

Management

If drugs/alcohol are the cause arrange supervision by relatives. Look for and treat organic illness – e.g. heart failure. Resist demands to have elderly patient taken away as an emergency. Admission may make the patient worse, but is indicated if patient lives alone and is unmanageable. Bed in psychogeriatric unit. Police have power to remove to a place of safety a patient found wandering.

Aggression/violence

Psychopaths who are often aggravated by drinks, drugs, etc. Epilepsy or schizophrenia may be cause.

Police may be needed before, with, or instead of the doctor. Plan approach with police (no heroics).

If *aggressive* person is a psychopath better not to label patient as ill. He/she should take responsibility for consequences of behaviour.

If *psychotic*, patient may need admission under sections 2 or 4.

If *violence is uncontrollable* give 200 mg i.m. promazine (Sparine) while patient is restrained by others.

Acutely psychotic

Schizophrenia. Schizophrenic patients are usually young, often lapsed from treatment. May have delusions, which may be paranoid.

Hallucinations, usually auditory. Behaviour may be bizarre.

Mania. Patient is excessively active in elated mood with no insight. Not usually violent unless restrained.

Depression. The patient may be guilt-ridden and retarded, some may be agitated. They cannot concentrate, have poor memory. There is a risk of suicide.

Management

If events out of control at home then arrange admission. Certify only if patient will not consent and if absolutely necessary. If agitated or excited give 200 mg i.m. promazine (Sparine).

Suicide threats/attempts

Hysterical. The patient is commonly a young woman who has taken tablets. She may be manipulative and action frequently follows family row/alcohol. Her attempt will have been well publicized.

Mentally ill. Generally among older patients. Methodical attempt. The attempt will not have been publicized.

Management

If an *overdose* has been taken the patient should be admitted to casualty.

A *threat* from a mentally ill patient must be taken seriously. Arrange for psychiatric opinion/admission.

A *threat* from an hysterical patient. Try to establish responsibility of patient for own actions and also responsibility of relatives and friends to supervise.

Anxiety/panic situational crisis

Neurosis. Usually a long-standing neurotic. May be the result of family crisis. Relatives and patient tend to be demanding. Hyperventilation is common. This is not really a medical emergency – make this clear.

Management

Calm firm handling essential. Do not give in to demands and manipulation.

Bereavement/grief

Uninhibited expressions of normal emotion are often regarded as 'illness' in our culture. Callers expect doctor to give drugs to suppress feelings.

Management

Putting an arm round the shoulders or holding the hand of the bereaved person does more than drugs and teaches the relatives what is required. At the very most, give some diazepam (Valium) for one or two nights though a stiff gin and tonic would probably do just as well.

Compulsory admission of psychiatric patients

England and Wales

Compulsion must be used only if the patient will not go voluntarily. Compulsion may be used when a patient suffers from a mental disorder that warrants detention in hospital when treatment is necessary for the patient's health or for the safety of the patient or others.

The DHSS recommends the use of section 2 (observation) if at all possible but in most GP emergencies section 4 (emergency) is more practical.

Section 4, *emergency, 72 hours.* One medical recommendation is needed. Applied for by approved social worker for nearest relative. Must state that using section 2 would cause unacceptable delay. Patient must be admitted within 24 hours, or earlier, of application or medical recommendation.

Section 2, *observation, 28 days.* Two medical recommendations necessary – one doctor with special psychiatric experience and one who has previous knowledge of the patient. Application by nearest relative or a social worker is needed. If the nearest relative objects social worker *cannot* apply. Nearest relatives are spouse; child; father; mother.

Procedure. Medical recommendation precedes the application. Arrange application by social worker if possible because most relatives would rather not be involved. You must arrange a bed with the hospital – completing an order does not guarantee a bed.

(Always keep a Section 4 form in your bag, then you are not dependent on the social worker.)

Scotland

In emergency use Section 31 of the Mental Health Act (Scotland) 1960.

One medical recommendation by doctor who has seen the patient that day necessary.

You must try to obtain consent of relative or mental officer: if not obtained you must state why. A patient can be detained for 7 days.

Northern Ireland

In emergency use admission form 3 of the Mental Health (Northern Ireland) Act 1961.

Part 1: Application by relative or social worker.
Part 2: Medical recommendation by doctor stating: when examined; clinical condition; why detention in hospital is needed and why informal admission is not suitable.

Patients can be detained for 7 days.

Acute vertigo

Vertigo is a definite loss of spatial orientation – usually with a feeling of rotation – and most emergency calls are for a first attack.

Sudden onset of vertigo is frightening. Patients usually complain of being dizzy or giddy; make sure you find out exactly what the patient means.

Telephone

Acute vertigo, especially with vomiting, is distressing and, unless it is a recurrent problem, is a good reason for an emergency consultation.

Assessment

In an emergency the doctor's primary task is to exclude serious disease of the ear or central nervous system (CNS). Often there is no cause.

Ears. Check for any evidence of active middle-ear infection. Discharge from the middle ear means invasive infection until proved otherwise. Refer urgently.

If you can provoke vertigo with sudden pressure down the line of the external auditory meatus with the ball of your finger, this will confirm your diagnosis.

Occasionally wax or debris may be the cause. Check the hearing – sensorineural deafness may indicate a tumour or auditory neuroma.

CNS. Examine CNS carefully. Any CNS signs or symptoms would make you suspect a central vascular lesion, tumour or, in a young person, multiple sclerosis.

Eyes – nystagmus. Nystagmus has two components: slow deviation of eyes and rapid return to midline. The slow component is towards the side of the lesion. Signs of unilateral nystagmus are: lack of a latent period, non-fatiguability and nystagmus in any plane apart from the horizontal. These signs should make you suspect a central cause.

CNS. Check for evidence of cerebrovascular insufficiency – carotid bruits and vertebrobasilar artery syndrome.

Management

If patient still has vertigo when seen give prochlorperazine 25 mg (Stemetil) i.m., or as a suppository. When the acute attack is over, give oral prochlorperazine or similar drug, for a few days.

If there is middle-ear infection, or any possibility of serious CNS disease, refer urgently.

Follow-up

See the patient 1–2 weeks later for review. If vertigo recurs, further evaluation will be necessary.

Eyes

Acutely painful and/or red eye

This is a common GP problem. If bilateral it is generally conjunctivitis. *Beware* the unilateral red/painful eye.

Loss of vision is possible from such conditions as herpetic keratitis or acute glaucoma. Careful evaluation: good lighting, loupe, sterile anaesthetic and fluorescein drops and an ophthalmoscope.

Telephone

See patient urgently if eye is definitely painful, rather than gritty, or if there is any loss of vision.

Assessment

See Table 19.1.

Management

- *Acute iritis* or *keratitis* – urgent ophthalmic opinion required.
- *Acute glaucoma* – refer and probably admit.
- *Large ulcer* or *dendritic ulcer*, or *herpes zoster* – refer for urgent ophthalmic opinion.
- *Small ulcer* on periphery or *minor abrasion*:
  - give cyclopentolate 0.5 per cent 1–2 drops;
  - apply chloramphenicol ointment;
  - apply pad and bandage; review in 24 hours.

Do not use steroid drops and *do not* pad conjunctivitis.

Arc eye

These are corneal flash burns due to ultraviolet light, usually caused by arc welding. Symptoms start several hours after exposure.

- Give amethocaine 1 per cent and cyclopentolate 0.5 per cent drops.
- Pad and bandage.
- Give oral analgesics.
- Review patient's condition in 48 hours.

Foreign bodies in eyes (see also page 158).

Take a careful history to determine if there is any possibility of a penetrating injury, e.g. metal grinding or the use of hammer and chisel.

Table 19.1 *Eye assessment chart*

Features	Acute conjunctivitis	Acute iritis	Acute glaucoma	Keratitis/corneal ulcer
Pain	Gritty rather than pain	Moderate Photophobia	Severe and radiating	Moderate
Discharge	Often pus	None	None	May occur
Visual disturbance	Smeared but no loss	Blurred	Gross with haloes	Blurred if area affected
Conjunctival injection	Peripheral	Around cornea	Diffuse	Around cornea or diffuse
Pupil/light reflex	Normal	Small, irregular, sluggish	Large, oval, fixed	Normal
Cornea	Clear	Clear or slightly hazy	Steamy	Ulcer or hazy patches
Intraocular pressure	Normal	Normal	High	Normal

Assessment

Give amethocaine 1 per cent drops to facilitate examination; fluorescein may be necessary to locate foreign body.

Management

If foreign body is large, deeply embedded or there is any possibility of a penetrating injury – send to ophthalmic casualty. Otherwise attempt removal with moist swab or the tip of a hypodermic needle. If successful, apply chloromycetin ointment. Pad eye and review in 24 hours. If unsuccessful, refer patient to ophthalmic casualty department.

Sudden loss of vision

This is frightening and all patients need to be seen urgently. Unilateral loss or a field of defect may have been present for some time, but patient may only just have noticed it.

Assessment

First determine whether or not vision has actually been lost – try to eliminate hysterical loss of vision.
- Is it longstanding? It is not uncommon for a patient with slowly developing cataract to realize suddenly that there is unilateral loss of vision and then to panic.

- Look for:
    – retinal artery occlusion – pale empty eyes;
    – retinal vein occlusion – congested with haemorrhages.
    – vitreous haemorrhage – blood obscures view of fundus.
    – retinal detachment – with field loss and dark bulge in retina.
- Consider the possibility of cranial arteritis or migraine.

Management

Any sudden and persistent loss of vision needs urgent referral. Often there is no remedy, but patient's anxiety needs relieving. Retinal detachment is most important because sight may be saved. Any small, sudden field loss, even if you cannot see a detachment on fundoscopy, needs *immediate* referral. Do not let the patient drive or undertake any exertion.

Alleged assault

Telephone

Advise if casualty/police should be involved rather than you. If visit is necessary to record injuries rather than for treatment, arrange to see patient at your convenience.

Management

Make detailed record of injuries. If injuries are serious send to casualty. If minor, treat as necessary.

Alleged indecent assault or rape

In these cases the police and a trained police surgeon ought to be involved. Strongly advise this from the onset. If you do see the patient then a lot of sympathy and tact is necessary. Do nothing which may confuse or destroy evidence.

Leave the gathering of evidence to a police surgeon unless you are suitably trained yourself.

WHAT TO DO WITH A DEAD BODY

Whether or not a death is expected it is reasonable and kind to visit to confirm death, give moral support and advice to relatives, and make sure about the circumstances of death.

Assessment

Diagnosis of death. Be careful, you will look silly if the patient wakes up later in the mortuary. Look for:

- Absent pulse.
- Absent heart sounds.
- Absent corneal and pupillary reflexes.
- Engorged retinal vessels.

If circumstances are suspicious, look for:

- Injuries.
- Strange attitudes or situation.
- Possibility of a poison.

Can you issue a certificate?

Yes – if you are satisfied death is natural and patient has been seen during the last 14 days.

No – if patient has not been seen during the last 14 days, if cause is unknown, if violent or accidental, or if connected with operation of anaesthetic.

The coroner must also be informed when death is: from industrial disease; in a patient with a pensioned disability; suicide; poisoning or due to drugs; due to want, exposure or neglect; or if any criticism of medical or nursing care is likely.

Management

Expected natural death. Confirm death and tell family to contact undertaker if this is desired. If only elderly or distressed spouse in house, you could do this.

Arrange for death certificate to be issued when convenient. Ask if cremation is intended and, if so, arrange for second medical certificate. If pacemaker is *in situ* – warn undertaker.

Unexpected death or if not seen in last 14 days. Confirm death and inform duty officer at police station. Give full details and your assessment of the situation. Do not allow the body to be removed.

If you are reasonably certain death was due to natural causes, the coroner may give you permission to issue an endorsed certificate (initialled in box A on reverse of form).

Chapter 20

Bread and butter medicine

Managing apparently minor disorders accounts for a large proportion of the GP's basic workload. As most of these conditions are hardly seen in hospital, or taught at medical school, trainees may initially experience difficulties in dealing with them. The brief notes which follow are designed to provide you with enough helpful, albeit dogmatic, information to allow you to cope satisfactorily until discussion with your trainer and further reading determine your individual views and management patterns.

Remember that although most of these conditions are trivial in a purely medical sense, they can provoke disproportionate anxiety and worry. Careful explanation is a vital part of management. Where explanation appears not to be readily accepted it is worth trying to discover what the patient feels or fears about the condition. Unless anxieties are ventilated and then allayed the consultation will not have a satisfactory outcome.

ACNE

Occurs as a reaction to sex hormone changes and affects four out of five teenagers. Blackheads and pimples on the face, back and chest look unsightly but in most cases they will clear up in the late teens or early twenties.

Frequent washing with soap and water and getting as much sunlight as possible will help; changing the diet will not and neither will squeezing the spots. Cosmetics should not be prohibited.

Anti-acne lotions or creams can be bought at the chemists or a benzoyl peroxide or retinoic acid-containing preparation prescribed. Severer cases may be helped by a 3-month course of oxytetracycline 250–500 mg twice a day.

Note: No tetracycline if there is any risk of pregnancy.

ALLERGIC RASHES

May be either a local contact dermatitis or a more generalized urticaria. Whatever the rash looks like it is likely to be sudden in onset and itchy. Urticaria may spread over large areas of the skin and may cause swelling (puffy eyes/difficulty in breathing). It generally clears up after a few days.

Identifying the cause and avoiding it may not be as easy as it sounds. An antihistamine may be prescribed for a few days if symptoms justify it.

Note: Contrary to popular belief an allergy can develop only to an allergen that the body has previously become sensitized to.

AMENORRHOEA

Best assumed to be caused by pregnancy until proved otherwise. Associated frequency, nausea or vomiting, faintness, breast soreness or tingling, sleepiness and constipation confirm the diagnosis without any need for pregnancy tests.

Note: Anxiety and emotional upset may well cause amenorrhoea and so may thyrotoxicosis.

ATHLETE'S FOOT

A fungal infection by no means confined to athletes. It starts between the toes, especially the little ones, with irritation and peeling of the skin which may spread to include the sole.

Keeping the feet clean and dry and avoiding tight-fitting footwear will help. Antifungal creams and powders may be prescribed or bought cheaply at the chemist and should be used regularly not just until irritation abates but until the skin between the toes returns completely to normal.

Note: Shoe dermatitis will not respond to fungicides.

BALANITIS

Presents with soreness, redness of the foreskin or glans and – often profuse – discharge. It should not be confused with a red ammoniacal foreskin from nappy rash or with paraphimosis. If it occurs in older males then venereal disease, diabetes and carcinoma of the penis should be excluded.

Any antiseptic cream may be used locally and, if infection looks severe, a penicillin may be prescribed. Recurrent infection associated with phimosis may necessitate circumcision.

Note: The foreskin does not usually retract until a child is 2–3 years old.

BALDNESS

Male pattern, which starts in the late teens and slowly progresses, is so common as not to be abnormal.

In women the hair thins mainly on the top of the head and total loss will not occur. Thinning may be caused by tight plaits or sleeping in rollers or, rarely, by anaemia or myxoedema. Temporary loss may follow pregnancy, stopping the pill or an illness with a high fever.

When there is fairly sudden onset of patchy loss (alopecia) the hair will, in most cases, regrow within 2–3 months though the larger the bald area the less likely it is that regrowth will be complete.

Note: There are no NHS prescribable scalp preparations that will affect the outcome. A private prescription for Regaine may if patient can afford it.

BELL'S PALSY

Refers to an isolated benign unilateral paralysis of the facial nerve. Onset is rapid and often accompanied by a dull ache or wooden feeling round the ear. The affected side of the face may be seen to have lost its expression and on smiling is drawn across to the unaffected side. Often the eyes cannot close completely. Sensory testing is normal. In severer cases there may be hyperacusis and loss of taste. In the absence of other symptoms indicating a more widespread neurological disease, otroscopic examination to exclude chronic middle-ear disease is all that is necessary.

With partial paralysis recovery will begin in 7–10 days and be complete in about 6 weeks. With total paralysis most people recover completely but a minority will not, though they may improve after 3 months or so. Simple analgesics, strict oral hygiene, taping the eyelid down at night, and regular gentle massaging of the affected muscles may help as may early high dose corticosteroid therapy (20 mg three times a day reducing by 5 mg daily).

Note: In rare bilateral cases check the urine for sugar.

BIRTH MARKS

May be *portwine stains*, which are present at birth as red, slightly raised areas; they do not spread further but persist throughout life without any improvement, or *strawberry naevi* which appear within the first week of life as a small red spot then rapidly enlarge, to become deep red and raised above the skin surface, until the age of 18 months after which they remain static until the age of 3 years when they start to shrink to disappear completely by 5 to 6 years.

There is no real treatment in either case though portwine stains especially can be cosmetically camouflaged with covering creams.

Note: Careful sympathetic explanation of the natural history is essential.

BLEPHARITIS

In its common form blepharitis is an outpost of dandruff from the scalp affecting the lid margins so that they become red, crusted and itchy. For effective treatment the dandruff must be controlled; crusts and discharge removed by cotton wool and water; and an antibiotic ointment (chloramphenicol) applied three times a day.

Note: Recurrence is highly likely.

BOILS

These start around a hair root then spread into the surrounding skin. They are usually single but may be multiple or recurrent.

Dry heat may be used to help pointing, when incision and drainage will be more effective in producing resolution than antibiotics. Incision of large boils may require a general anaesthetic.

Note: Recurrent boils may be due to diabetes but are more likely to be due to reinfection by staphylococci from the nares, genitalia or axillae.

BUNIONS

Typically develop in middle-aged women as the big toe is pushed permanently outwards, probably by ill-fitting shoes, and a bursa develops over the medial aspect of the first metatarsophalangeal joint.

A chiropodist may be able to help but surgical treatment is likely to be necessary in severe, painful cases.

Note: Infection of the overlying bursa is not uncommon.

CARPAL TUNNEL SYNDROME

Mostly occurs in overweight, middle-aged housewives who, by constant flexing and extending of the wrist, damage the median nerve within the carpal tunnel. A minority of cases arise as a feature of an underlying disease, e.g. old fracture, acromegaly, myxoedema, oedema (especially in pregnancy when it will resolve after delivery).

Pain – which may radiate up the arm – tingling and numbness are felt in the hand and fingers in the median nerve distribution. Attacks are most common at night, often waking the patient, and are relieved by shaking the hand or hanging the affected arm out of the bed.

Cases with severe or recurrent symptoms or any objective signs of neurological deficit in the hands must be treated with early surgical decompression. For milder symptoms relief may be gained by resting the hand and wrist (a resting night splint helps); a short course of a non-steroidal anti-inflammatory drug; weight reduction; and a diuretic if symptoms are worse premenstrually or aggravated by oedema from other causes.

Note: The adductor pollicis is the only thenar eminence muscle spared.

CATARRH

Normally means a more than usual amount of secretions coming from the nose or bronchi. It may result from an oversensitive mucosa reacting to irritants, including dust and pollen, or infection. Thick yellow or green nasal discharge is usual.

In the absence of a treatable cause antibiotics are unlikely to give anything other than temporary relief as are nasal decongestant drops.

Note: First find out what the patient means by catarrh.

CHICKENPOX

Highly infectious, usually mild, illness with an incubation period of 15–18 days and period of infectivity from one day before to 6 days after the rash. The rash is usually the first sign of infection and the vesicles come in crops, crusting within 7 days of arising.

If there is no chest, ear or sinus infection then treatment is purely symptomatic. Calamine lotion may be applied to itchy spots.

Note: One attack confers lifelong immunity.

COLDS

Common and usually self-treated. If patients come to the doctor it may be for a sick note; examination to exclude complications (babies are often brought because of worries that the cold has 'gone to the chest'); or in the hope or expectation of a prescription.

Unless sinusitis, bronchitis or otitis media are present no prescription is necessary though babies may benefit from nasal drops (ephedrine 0.5 per cent 15 minutes before feeds) and chronic bronchitics etc. from early antibiotics. General advice about symptomatic treatment should be given to everyone.

Note: Non-prescribing for simple self-limiting conditions encourages patients to treat themselves the next time.

COLD SORES

Caused by the herpes simplex virus which lies dormant in the skin repeatedly flaring up to produce, usually at the same site, painful sores on the lips, nose or cheeks.

Healing normally occurs within 10 days though surgical spirit or toilet water applied 3–4 hourly may speed this up. Ice applied to the sores has also been reported to be effective.

Note: If severe and recurrent, acyclovir (Zovirax) cream used as soon as symptoms begin may be effective though likely effect must be balanced against expense.

COLIC (3 MONTHS OR EVENING)

Attacks usually begin within the first 15 days of life and recur nightly until at from 10–16 weeks they resolve completely. During attacks the baby's face becomes red, he draws his legs up, emits piercing screams and cannot be comforted. After 2–20 minutes pain suddenly ceases though regular occurrences last until about 10–11 at night when sleep supervenes.

Gentle pressure or massage of the abdomen, placing baby on his tummy and giving a breast or bottle to suck may all give some relief during an attack.

Note: Reassurance and explanation go a long way to helping the mother to cope.

CONJUNCTIVITIS

The commonest cause of red eyes and this condition is characterized by generalized conjunctival injection; discharge, most noticeable on waking; grittiness, rather than pain; and, if present, very mild photophobia. Visual acuity is unchanged and the pupil is normal.

Antibiotic drops (chloramphenicol) used 2–3-hourly, or more frequently if necessary, should be prescribed and the discharge kept clear with cotton wool and water. The eye should not be padded.

Note: Unilateral conjunctivitis should not be diagnosed so readily as bilateral conjunctivitis.

CRADLE CAP

Tends to appear first at about 1 month of age and clears up at 6 months. The yellow brown greasy scalp scaling is very common and usually mild though occasionally it may be severe with thick yellow lumps rather than scales.

A mild keratolytic, e.g. cetrimide (Cetavlex) cream should be applied at night and shampooed out the next morning with a simple shampoo.

Note: Hair growth will not be affected in any way.

DANDRUFF

If dry, white, scaly and present for long periods, may be the only evidence of a seborrhoeic tendency. Severe scalp scaling may also be caused by psoriasis (patchy with palpable lesions) or atopic eczema and ichthyosis (past history and evidence of flexural lesions elsewhere on body).

Mild cases respond to detergent shampoos while severer dry scaling will be helped by selenium sulphide (Lenium, Selsun). These shampoos should be advised but not prescribed, though for psoriatic or eczematous scalps Polytar shampoo or Betnovate scalp application may be.

DYSMENORRHOEA

Most often affects young women and may start a day or two before the bleeding. Malaise, headache, nausea may also occur and there may be a link with constipation. It is not a sign of disease but if it is severe or a new symptom a vaginal examination should be carried out.

Sufferers should be advised to continue with all normal physical activities; avoid constipation at period time; and to try to resolve any contributory emotional problems. Soluble aspirin is a useful analgesic though if pain is still severe a non-steroidal anti-inflammatory agent may be prescribed.

Note: This is one condition greatly relieved by the pill.

EARACHE

Associated with an upper respiratory infection and a red drum is caused by otitis media. A normal drum but tender pinna would suggest an external meatal boil while intermittent pain with a normal ear suggests a dental origin. Hard wax may be the cause but it is wise to check the drum after syringing.

In all cases simple analgesics should be advised. Dry heat may help a boil to point while antibiotics are necessary in most, but certainly not all, cases of otitis media. Amoxycillin (Amoxil) is the antibiotic of choice and is effective if taken for at least 3 days.

Note: Babies cannot complain of earache and so rely on you to make the diagnosis for them.

ECZEMA

Caused by primary irritants and allergy, eczema may be easily diagnosed on the basis of the distribution of the rash and an adequate history (including occupation and hobbies). Prevention of further exposure of the skin to the substance responsible for the reaction is of paramount importance. One per cent hydrocortisone cream applied 3 or 4 times a day will help though sometimes a more potent preparation may be needed.

Atopic eczema affects about 10 per cent of children and in the vast majority it will clear permanently in childhood. It is usually mild and begins after the age of 3 months, most often affecting flexures then face, neck and hands. Parents must be warned that exacerbations are characteristic and that creams like 1 per cent hydrocortisone are suppressive not curative. Stronger steroids should be used only in short courses if the eczema proves refractory.

Note: This is not a contraindication to any vaccination.

ENURESIS

Not a disease, but delayed development of bladder control. At 3 years 75 per cent of children are dry by night; at 6 years 92 per cent and at 12 years virtually all. In less than 3 per cent of primary enuretics there will be an underlying organic abnormality, e.g. mental retardation, lesion of the lower spinal cord, urinary tract abnormalities. Secondary enuresis developing after the child has achieved control may be due to the onset of urinary infection, diabetes or epilepsy but it is far more likely to be caused by a sudden emotional disturbance.

After the age of 5–6 treatment may be justified. Parents should be advised *to praise and reward* for dry nights; empty bladder before bed; lift as late as possible and be first one up in morning, and *not* to scold, blackmail or threaten, comment or tease about wet nights, restrict fluid intake, or increase salt in food. A chart of wet/dry nights allows the true frequency of wetting to be assessed, imipramine 25 mg at night will help high frequency wetters within a week and may reduce family tensions but has a high relapse rate; a pad and buzzer alarm will produce a long-term cure in 80 per cent of cases.

Note: Urinalysis and mid-stream urine specimen should be examined on presentation and if there is any recurrence.

EPISTAXIS

This comes predominantly from local trauma-related causes. Most cases are dealt with at home using simple first aid. Active bleeding should be treated with even and firm pressure applied to the anterior nasal septum by pinching the nostrils closed between thumb and forefinger. While the patient mouth breathes pressure is maintained for at least 5 minutes. Careful examination of the nose (using an auriscope) is best carried out when no bleeding is taking place.

Mild recurrent bleeds associated with nasal crusting may be helped by topical use of soft paraffin three times a day to soften the discharge, and localized nasal infection may be treated by an antibiotic cream. Frequent recurrences may need ENT referral for cautery to Little's area.

Note: Severe or recurrent bleeding warrants a full blood count.

FLAT FEET

Normal when a child starts to stand because the medial arch does not develop until the second or third year of life. After this age if the feet are still flat but are painfree with normal mobility and muscle power no treatment is necessary, though insoles may help shoe wear.

Feet that are painful, stiff or hypermobile, and weak or spastic may be part of a generalized condition, e.g. cerebral palsy, or indicate a local bony or inflammatory problem that needs diagnosis and treatment.

Note: Getting a child to stand on tiptoe will accentuate the medial arch.

FLEAS

Fleas generally drop off domestic pets on to furniture and carpets. A typical bite is urticarial with a central punctum and surrounding flare and may develop into quite a large blister. Bites tend to occur on exposed areas (below the knee, arms, hands) and discrete papules may persist for some months.

Furniture and carpets should be treated with an insecticide containing pyrethrum; pets should be treated by the vet; and antihistamines may be prescribed to relieve irritation.

Note: Persisting papules are often not suspected of being flea bites.

FOREIGN BODY IN THE EAR

Rarely causes damage comparable to that caused by ill-advised attempts at extraction. Some foreign bodies, e.g. paper, may be easily removed by syringing or blunt forceps but if the patient is not likely to be cooperative and quite still and if the doctor is not experienced in using a blunt right-angled probe (passed beyond foreign body and gently withdrawn) and head mirror then referral to casualty or ENT is indicated.

Note: Filling the ear with water will kill a live insect and give much relief.

FOREIGN BODY IN THE EYE

Demands a careful history to exclude any possibility of a penetrating injury, e.g. from metal grinding, use of hammer and chisel. If penetration was possible, the eye injured, or the foreign body deeply embedded in the cornea then the patient should be referred direct to casualty. If none of the problems are present 1 per cent amethocaine drops should be used for pain relief to allow careful eye examination (including subtarsal area). The foreign body may be removed with a moist cotton wool swab or, if practised, an embedded particle may be removed using a hypodermic needle.

Once removed, the eye should be stained with fluorescein to assess damage, chloramphenicol drops instilled, eye padded for 12 hours, and the patient seen again in 48 hours to recheck the cornea.

Note: If there is any possibility of penetration – even if the patient feels only vaguely that something is in the eye – this is an ocular emergency.

FOREIGN BODY IN THE NOSE

If not removed by forcible nose blowing and not easily seen and grasped by forceps or got behind by angled probe then refer direct to ENT. Definite risk of inhalation so immediate referral necessary.

Note: Consider this in any child with foul-smelling unilateral discharge or persistent bad breath.

GLANDULAR FEVER

Generally affects teenagers and though not very infectious may develop 1–2 weeks after contact with a case. Most patients feel ill with a swinging temperature and a very sore throat which may persist for weeks associated with lymphadenopathy. A rash or jaundice may develop and while children tend to recover quickly adults may feel below par for weeks after an attack.

A Monospot test will confirm the diagnosis. No treatment, other than plenty of fluids and regular simple analgesics, will have any effect.

Note: Suspect this in any teenager with a severe sore throat not responding to penicillin.

HALITOSIS

Tends to be a temporary state that will resolve naturally. If persistent it is likely to be the result of personal habits, e.g. stale tobacco smoke, spicy, garlic-laden foods, alcohol, poor dental care. It is seldom caused by any serious disease though it may be associated with chronic nasal and chest infections.

Advice may be given on personal habits or a visit to the dentist suggested. If ENT examination reveals purulent postnasal or nasal discharge an antibiotic may be prescribed.

Note: Most smells come from anaerobic bacteria so metronidazole (Flagyl) might well be the antibiotic of choice. In children exclude a nasal foreign body.

HAY FEVER

A grass-pollen allergy causing coryza-like symptoms, conjunctival irritation and even wheezing in sensitive individuals seasonally from late May to mid-July. A common problem, it usually begins in the teens and recurs annually for 5–15 years until natural resolution occurs. Diagnosis presents few problems – but non-grass pollen allergies are less dramatic in their presentation and occur at different times of the year – and is simply based on history.

Symptom severity is proportional to atmospheric pollen count and sufferers should avoid walking through long grass, camping, car or train journeys with open windows, and house windows open on hot, humid, windy days, though complete avoidance of pollen is impractical. Other than these measures, mild symptoms need no treatment beyond the wearing of sunglasses and the liberal use of hankies.

Social factors, e.g. type of employment, driving, important forthcoming events, are as important as the severity of symptoms in deciding treatment. Vasoconstrictor nose drops are useful in an emergency; antihistamines may need to be changed around to find the one most suitable for a particular patient or when tolerance develops; topical disodium cromoglycate and steroids are costly and not always well tolerated; systemic steroids may be justified for severe symptoms or to tide the patient over an important event.

Note: It is well worth taking time initially to explain the aetiology of the condition and self-help measures available.

HYPERHIDROSIS

In hot humid weather hyperhidrosis may produce the itchy rash of prickly heat, though when patients complain of excess perspiration they are usually referring to local sweating. Very sweaty feet macerate the skin and give an unpleasant smell. Very sweaty axillae and palms are usually caused by emotional tension and typically affect female teenagers.

Feet can be helped by avoiding rubber-soled shoes, wearing sandals wherever possible and soaking the soles of the feet in 3 per cent formalin solution for 5–10 minutes each night. Prickly heat is helped by wearing little and loose clothing, using fans to cool the skin surface and limiting activity to reduce sweating. Axillary sweating is helped by wearing sleeveless dresses, not overusing underarm deodorants and trying to reduce tension and stress. In severe cases application of a 20 per cent solution of aluminium chloride hexahydrate in absolute alcohol painted on nightly for one week is effective though hydrocortisone ointment may be needed for irritant skin reaction. Excision of apocrine gland areas may be necessary.

Note: Heat-induced sweating is normal and requires no treatment.

IMPETIGO

An epidermal infection by *Staphylococcus aureus* or a streptococcus. Superficial spreading yellow crusts are usually found on the face and hands. Circinate lesions with less distinct crusting and a clearly defined spreading edge may occur. Satellite lesions are common.

Careful personal hygiene is necessary to stop the spread and a topical antibiotic, e.g. sodium fusidate (Fucidin) should be used four times a day until all signs of the disorder are cleared. A course of penicillin may be given if the condition is extensive or recurrent.

Note: Many schools insist on keeping children away until their impetigo has completely cleared up. This is unnecessary and may be avoided if the doctor confines his/her diagnosis to 'a skin infection'.

INFLUENZA

Term used by both doctors and patients for feverish upper respiratory tract infections seldom due to any specific virus. Malaise, fever, cough, coryza, aching and sweating last 2–3 days and are followed by gradual improvement. Most cases are uncomplicated and benign but in epidemic influenza there is a case fatality rate of 1 in 500 (mainly in the elderly).

General measures are all that is necessary unless secondary bacterial infection supervenes. Antibiotics should be used sooner rather than later in the elderly and patients with chronic cardiac or respiratory conditions.

Note: Malaria cases are often wrongly diagnosed as flu.

INGROWING TOENAILS

Mainly confined to the big toenails of teenage boys. Medical advice is usually sought when infection develops in the skin round the nail.

Mild infections can be treated by antibiotic creams while more severe infections will need an oral antibiotic. Good foot hygiene, going barefoot or in sandals wherever possible, and cutting the toenail at a right angle to the long axis of the toe may help. Cutting away the ingrowing part of the nail may be necessary.

Severe or persistent cases may require surgical referral for removal of the nail.

Note: Your trainer may have his/her own minor operation for dealing with this problem.

INSECT BITES AND STINGS

Mainly from bees and wasps, will present because of pain, swelling or fears of local infection. A bee sting can be scraped out with a finger nail and the site should be cleaned with antiseptic. Soluble aspirin is an effective analgesic and unless swelling is marked and spreading – when an antihistamine may be prescribed – or secondary infection appears to be present – when an antibiotic may be needed – the patient should be advised that symptoms will resolve within 2–3 days.

Note: A few people are hypersensitive to bee or wasp venom and may be killed by a single sting.

INSOMNIA

Not a disease per se but it may be a symptom of physical or psychological disorder. Most often it is a normal sleep pattern variation which for some reason has become unacceptable.

Any underlying disease should be treated in its own right, e.g. depression with antidepressants; pain with analgesics. When there is no underlying disease, explanation that sleep needs differ from person to person and from time to time and will sort themselves out should be given. It is worth saying that an elderly person averages only 4–5 hours sleep a night and that catnapping during the day is just as good as sleep at night. Simple advice on improving sleep quality can be given, namely, a regular routine at night with a walk or hot bath, hot milky drink and a quiet book; no television or work in the bedroom; comfortable bed and surroundings.

If prescribed at all, hypnotics should be prescribed for only a short course and it should be made clear to the patient that when the tablets are finished no more will be forthcoming.

Note: The best way to avoid hypnotic dependence is by not prescribing in the first place.

INTOEING

Where the toes turn in, or one leg is thrown around the other, or the child falls over his own feet, is fairly common when walking begins. In most cases the cause lies above the knee so that the foot is normal and the child walks with the whole leg turned in and the knees facing a little towards each other. This nearly always corrects itself by the age of 6 and only if it is still severe then or appears for the first time after then would an orthopaedic opinion be needed.

Metatarsus varus, where the forefoot turns inward relative to the hindfoot, is usually recognized before the child starts to walk. Eight out of nine cases will correct themselves without treatment by the age of 3. Severe or persistent cases may need an orthopaedic opinion.

Note: Waiting to make sure the abnormality will not correct by itself does not make it any more difficult to treat later.

KNOCK KNEES

Symmetrically present, to some degree, in 75 per cent of 2–4½ year-olds. In 99 cases out of 100 this is a normal variation and will correct itself without treatment by the age of 7 years.

Pronounced asymmetry, short stature, an intermalleolar separation (measured with the child lying down) of 3½ inches or condition uncorrected by 10–11 years would warrant orthopaedic opinion.

Note: No damage will be caused by waiting for a child to grow out of mild knock knees and seeking further opinion only if it does not.

LARYNGITIS

This condition, with hoarse cough and hoarse or lost voice, is easily diagnosed. Symptoms may be part of a viral upper respiratory tract infection in which case general measures, including resting the voice, are all that is necessary and most patients will recover fully within 3–7 days. If there is evidence of sinusitis or severe systemic upset a broad spectrum antibiotic should be prescribed.

Note: Any hoarseness persisting for more than three weeks demands urgent ENT referral for laryngoscopy.

LICE

Seen mostly in children's heads, where the main symptom is itching. They are contagious and the eggs laid close to the scalp become attached to growing hairs and develop into nits (small white specks firmly attached to the hair shafts). All members of the family should be treated at the same time by washing the hair, then applying malathion 0.5 per cent solution liberally, leaving for 12 hours, then shampooing the scalp again and combing the wet hair with a fine-tooth comb. Treatment is best repeated in one week.

Pubic lice are treated in the same way (without fine-tooth combing) but if found the question of whether other venereal diseases are present or not should be raised.

Note: Nits cannot be brushed off, whereas dandruff can.

LUMPS AND BUMPS

Those proffered for an opinion include lipomas, lymph nodes, papillomas, sebaceous cysts, ganglia, warts, moles, boils, rodent ulcers and so on. Presentation is either for reassurance that nothing serious is amiss or for removal of the offending lump on cosmetic or other grounds.

If the patient wishes it, or if there is any suspicion whatsoever of malignancy, removal should be arranged either within the practice or at a hospital outpatient clinic.

Note: Multiple lipomas may be neurofibromas.

MEASLES

Highly infectious with an incubation period of 10–14 days followed by 3–4 days of feverish upper respiratory tract infection symptoms before the development of the characteristic maculopapular rash. Pyrexia may persist for the first 2–3 days of the rash after which the child's condition rapidly improves. The infectious stage lasts for 5 days before the rash appears to 5 days after the temperature is back to normal.

Acute otitis media and chest infection are the main complications requiring antibiotic treatment. Management otherwise is on general lines with plenty of fluids, 4-hourly paracetamol, bed rest if the child desires it, and possibly an antihistamine cough medicine, e.g. Phenergan (Promethazine HCl), at night for its sedative effect.

Note: During a measles epidemic it is wise to say to all parents that their child's cold may be prodromal measles.

MEIBOMIAN CYST

Granuloma occurring in a Meibomian gland giving rise to a chronic painless (unless infection develops) swelling usually situated at some distance from the lid margin. Eyes referral may be required for incision and curettage if spontaneous resolution does not occur.

Note: Pain implies abscess formation.

MENOPAUSE

Retrospectively diagnosed occurs on average at age 51 when women may already be experiencing anxieties about future functioning, doubts about their attractiveness and sexuality, and fears of approaching old age. Sudden hormone changes may be associated with unpleasant symptoms, many of which are coincidental and as likely to be helped by placebo as oestrogen. The symptoms of vasomotor instability (flushes, sweats and flush-induced insomnia) and of urogenital atrophy may be oestrogen-deficiency related. Only a minority of women will feel that their menopausal symptoms warrant a medical opinion.

A sympathetic ear in itself may be therapeutic and avoidance of stress and alcohol will decrease flushing. Atrophic vaginitis may be helped by using KY jelly for lubrication during intercourse or by oestrogen-containing creams. Vasomotor symptoms if severe may be temporarily allayed by ethinyloestradiol 10 micrograms three times a day for 2–3 months (if longer then a combined preparation). There are many arguments for and against long-term hormone replacement therapy which are beyond the scope of this book.

Note: Contraception is recommended for 2 years after the presumed last period if the woman is below 50 and for one year if she is over 50.

MOLES

Moles, or pigmented naevi, are not all present at birth and may appear in childhood. Every adult has some – on average 15–20. Their importance lies in the very small chance they have of developing into malignant melanoma. Sudden enlargement, alteration in pigmentation of the lesion or the surrounding skin, and bleeding or ulceration of the lesion should all raise the suspicion of malignancy.

Other reasons for surgical excision are cosmetic and where the lesion is prominently situated on part of the skin which is subject to trauma from clothing.

Note: No other forms of treatment should be attempted.

MOUTH ULCERS

Usually multiple, sore, and shallow, about 2–10 mm in diameter and found on the tongue, floor of the mouth and inside of the cheeks.

These aphthous ulcers each take about 4–10 days to heal and the tendency to develop them persists for many years. No treatment is effective, but avoiding smoking, hot food and ill-fitting dentures may help as may good dental hygiene.

Single persistent ulcers may be from a rough tooth or denture though the possibility of malignancy should be considered.

Note: Soluble aspirin gargled then swallowed is as helpful as anything else.

MUMPS

Essentially a benign disease and even in complicated cases (orchitis, oophoritis, pancreatitis, aseptic meningitis), complete recovery with no sequelae is the rule. Incubation period is 18–21 days with the patient being infectious for 2–3 days before the swelling occurs and remaining so until the glands have returned to normal size.

Mild constitutional upset may be experienced for a day or two before and after salivary gland (mainly parotid) enlargement appears. Swelling is often better seen than felt and characteristically one parotid pushes the earlobe upward and forwards while obliterating the groove between the ramus of the jaw and the mastoid process.

Children are little affected and need no more than simple analgesics and a good fluid intake. Adults may feel the need for bed rest. Orchitis symptoms can be dramatically relieved by a short course of prednisolone (15 mg four times a day for four days).

Note: Although children with mumps should be kept away from adults there is a strong case for trying to ensure that other children catch the infection. Mumps now is preventible with MMR vaccine.

NAPPY RASH

Primary irritation of the skin by prolonged contact with wet or dirty nappies, aggravated by the moisture-retaining action of plastic pants, characteristically spares the skin creases and folds. The inflamed and broken skin easily becomes secondarily infected with candida (isolated spots in the nappy area or failure to respond to simple measures suggests this) or pyogenic bacteria. Spread into the creases or out of the nappy area may occur in an atopic baby as a smoother, more shiny rash than usual or as napkin psoriasis.

Nappies should be changed as soon as possible after they become wet or soiled. The baby's bottom should be washed and thoroughly dried before being left exposed for as long as possible before a new nappy, with liner, is put on. Plastic pants should be avoided until the rash clears. In mild cases a simple emollient ointment such as zinc and castor oil may be used but where secondary infection is suspected an ointment like Nystaform HC (contains nystatin, clioquinol and hydrocortisone) should be used three times a day. Oral or maternal thrush should be treated at the same time.

Note: Mother must understand that her care of the baby is the single most important factor in effecting a cure.

NASAL POLYPS

Follow either prolonged allergic rhinitis or chronic sinusitis and present with nasal obstruction, mouth breathing, snoring and loss of sense of smell. The polyp is a round, shiny grey obstruction which can be seen filling the nasal passage.

Treatment is surgical but recurrence after removal is likely.

Note: Mechanical obstruction is unlikely to be helped by any medication, although Beconase nasal spray may give some relief.

NIGHT CRAMPS

Precipitated by random muscle contraction or voluntary stretching movements are quite a common cause of sleep disturbance in the elderly.

Keeping the bedclothes loose may help as may quinine sulphate 125 to 300 mg at night. Nevertheless, stretching exercises (stand 1 metre from wall, heels on floor, control forward tilt by hands outstretched onto wall. Stretch until moderate pulling sensation experienced in calves for 10 seconds then come back to upright posture to relax for 10 seconds before repeating. Continue for 5–10 minutes three times a day until cured) will cure most cases within a month or two.

Note: Although explaining the exercises may initially take longer than prescribing, the time and money saved by not having to prescribe repeatedly more than compensates.

OBESITY

A topic about which several books have been written. For practical purposes it is sufficient to say that group therapy (Weight Watchers, etc.) is far more likely to achieve sustained weight reduction than the GP. It is worth giving enthusiasts a diet sheet and offering to reweigh them in 1–2 weeks but the importunings of 'yo-yo' fatties for prescriptions for diuretics or appetite suppressants should be firmly resisted.

Note: A well-trained practice nurse can deal with the practice's dieters as well as any doctor.

OTITIS EXTERNA

Presents with itching or irritation, discharge and, possibly, pain in the ears. It is usually a recurrent problem which will flare up if the external canal becomes wet.

Treatment with combination antibacterial/steroid drops, e.g. Locorten-Vioform four times a day, will often be all that is needed. If infection is severe an oral broad-spectrum antibiotic should also be given.

Note: If infection persists despite treatment check the urine for sugar.

OUT-TOEING

Charlie Chaplin-like walk is quite common within the first 2 years of life. It may be more pronounced on one side than the other and although most cases correct spontaneously with time it is important to make sure that the hips and spine are normal.

Note: This may make the child appear to have very flat feet.

PILES

May present with fresh bleeding at the end of defaecation, prolapse, irritation and itching, and pain. If untreated, spontaneous improvement will occur but recurrence is likely particularly if constipation is not avoided. However strong a past history the GP should not be deterred from performing a rectal examination in any adult with symptoms of piles to try to exclude carcinoma of rectum. If there is any suspicion of bowel cancer, sigmoidoscopy should be arranged.

Simple suppositories or creams such as Anusol or Anusol HC will help soothe the pain and discomfort. A high-fibre diet will help avoid constipation and good anal hygiene will help decrease irritation. Recurrent problems may justify injection or haemorrhoidectomy.

Note: Creams containing local anaesthetics may ease anal pain initially but as they act as potent sensitizers may cause more irritation in the end.

PITYRIASIS ROSEA

Usually begins with the solitary herald patch. This is on the trunk and is a reddish brown annular scaly patch. Within 1–2 weeks other lesions appear on the trunk and tend to remain confined to the vest and pants area. These lesions may be oval macules, with their long axes in the lines of cleavage of the skin, or pink papules.

Apart from occasional irritation the disease is symptomless and will clear within 2–3 months of onset.

Note: Once the patient has been assured of the benign self-limiting nature of the disease no active treatment is necessary.

PREMENSTRUAL SYNDROME

Refers to a wide range of psychiatric and somatic symptoms occurring in the 10–14 days before menstruation, and resolving for at least 7 days after. Those most often described are irritability, depression, exhaustion, panic, painful or tender breasts, oedema, stomach ache, nausea and headache. The basic cause is unknown though psychological factors play a part and it seems fair to assume some direct or indirect hormone influences are at work.

Sympathetic, clear explanation of why symptoms are being experienced coupled with reassurance that they are part of a normal cycle and not a disease process may help. Symptoms of fluid retention may be relieved by a thiazide diuretic; symptoms of anxiety may be helped by a mild tranquilizer; and headaches and other aches and pains may be relieved by simple analgesics. Any drugs given will excite a significant placebo response and vitamin B_6 may be used as a cheap, safe placebo. In severe cases not helped by simpler treatment, progesterone suppositories or pessaries (Cyclogest) are worth considering.

Note: There is no doubt that premenstrual changes exist but their existence does not imply that they are due to disease or that they need treatment.

PSORIASIS

Common skin disorder of unknown aetiology. It usually appears between the ages of 15 and 30 and shows different degrees of activity. Over a third of cases will remit, either spontaneously or after treatment, but the length of remission is variable.

Clinical diagnosis is generally easy. The classical lesion is a red, raised, scaly (white or silvery) plaque with sharply demarcated edges. Knees, elbows, sacrum and scalp are the most common sites. Pitted, hyperkeratotic or onycholytic nails may occur.

Patients should be told that psoriasis is: not contagious; not a sign of internal disease; not going to leave scars or marks when it clears; likely to remit (unpredictably); likely to be helped by sunshine. They should also understand that although treatment may improve the condition there is no permanent cure available. For those who want treatment, local applications of coal tar or dithranol preparations should be tried first. Topical steroids are indicated for new lesions, psoriasis in the groins, axillae and face, and for chronic plaques.

Note: Although psoriasis cannot be cured the GP can still do a lot to help.

RAYNAUD'S DISEASE

In its mild form, this disease usually affects women. Digital artery spasm in cold weather makes the fingers go dead and white. After minutes or hours the circulation returns accompanied by pain and flushing of the affected fingers. There is no specific treatment. Cigarette smoking should be avoided and the hands kept as warm as possible at all times.

Note: Raynaud's disease that is secondary to use of vibrating tools, collagen diseases, severe anaemia, etc. is a more serious condition.

RINGWORM

Fungi are mostly transmitted from person to person though they may be acquired from cats, dogs and cattle.

Ringworm of the groin (*Tinea cruris*) starts with erythema and maceration of the skin and spreads out in an annular pattern with a raised red scaly margin. Perspiration should be avoided as far as possible and topical preparations, e.g. Whitfield's ointment, clotrimazole (Canestan), should be used. If inflammation is severe, hydrocortisone 1 per cent may help. If lesions are chronic then oral griseofulvin 500 mg daily for one month may be needed.

Ringworm of the body (*Tinea corporis*) characteristically forms a ring with an active edge and no clearing in the centre. Topical antifungals should be used but if infection does not clear griseofulvin may be needed.

Note: Household pets may need to be checked by a vet.

RUBELLA

Rubella has an incubation period of 10–21 days before maculopapular rash, suboccipital lymphadenopathy and mild fever develop. Symptoms last 2–4 days and patients are infectious 5 days before and 5 days after the rash. Clinical diagnosis is notoriously inaccurate.

Maternal rubella in pregnancy is associated with congenital abnormalities. If infection develops in the first 3–4 months of pregnancy then there is only a 1 in 3 chance of a completely normal child being born and termination should be considered.

Presentation of a patient who fears she has contracted rubella in early pregnancy is not uncommon. Pregnancy should be confirmed and rubella antibody titre estimated (over 80 per cent of women of childbearing age are immune). If there is no detectable rubella HI antibody a second specimen should be taken 7–10 days after the onset of any rubella-like illness or 30 days after the last day of contact if no illness develops. Seroconversion indicates rubella.

If antibodies are detected in serum taken within 10 days of contact the patient can be regarded as immune. Antibodies detected in serum taken more than 10 days after contact may be from a developing or remote infection. A repeat titre is necessary and a rise would indicate current infection while a static low titre would exclude recent rubella.

Note: Intrapractice screening and vaccination can eliminate the risk of congenital rubella.

SCABIES

Highly contagious and most often acquired by handholding or sharing a bed with an infected person. There is often a positive family history. Generalized irritation when going to bed at night is usually the presenting symptom with a rash developing later. Burrows on the hands or deep, red papules on the buttocks or genitalia are diagnostic though by the time the patient presents there is also usually a generalized excoriated papular urticarial rash.

Treatment consists of two applications of benzyl benzoate lotion to all members of the affected household (gamma benzene hexachloride in a 1 per cent cream is preferable for children). The lotion must be applied to all the skin surface from the neck to the soles of the feet. The patient should be warned that irritation may well persist for 1–2 weeks after successful treatment and that genital papules may persist for months.

Note: Suspect scabies in anyone whose itchy rash is worse at night.

SHINGLES

Like chickenpox, shingles is caused by the herpes zoster virus. Older people are generally affected and present with pain (often severe) felt unilaterally in the affected cutaneous segment. Between 2 and 14 days later one or more blotchy red patches appear, to be followed in 24 hours by the characteristic vesicles. Vesicles may persist for up to 5 weeks and in 5 per cent of cases will be followed by postherpetic neuralgia.

Trigeminal involvement with its associated corneal ulceration and other eye complications demands ophthalmic management. Strong analgesics may be needed, though pain can be rapidly relieved by a short course of prednisolone. Postherpetic neuralgia is commoner in elderly and debilitated patients. In these patients it is worth considering the use of idoxuridine or acyclovir (Herpid or Zovirax). Their use is not justified routinely.

Note: Severe pain in the chest or abdomen occurring before the rash develops may cause diagnostic confusion.

SINUSITIS

Most commonly affects the maxillary sinus. Clinical features include tenderness over the inflamed sinus, pus in the middle meatus and postnasal space, and some degree of constitutional upset.

Decongestants and analgesics help though antibiotics should be used sooner rather than later, particularly if frontal or ethmoidal sinuses seem to be involved.

Note: Sinusitis may present as upper jaw toothache.

SOILING

Soiling or persisting diarrhoea in children demands a rectal examination as impacted faeces will often be found. Initial treatment with glycerine suppositories or Microlax enema should be followed by regular laxative use coupled with toilet training to try to resolve the problem.

Note: Neither paediatricians nor child psychiatrists can easily help the encopretic child.

SORE THROATS

Caused by viruses in up to 80 per cent of cases and clinical signs correlate poorly with the aetiological agent. Plenty of fluids and simple analgesics should be advised with penicillin best reserved for patients with a moderate degree of constitutional upset and no other symptoms suggestive of a viral upper respiratory tract infection. Throat swabs will rarely influence either management or outcome.

Note: The worst-looking throats may well be glandular fever.

SNORING

Tends to have an adverse effect on everyone except the snorer. Kinking of the trachea by a sagging chin may be an aetiological factor and wearing a cervical collar (a rolled-up newspaper wrapped in a headscarf) at night might help.

Note: If the worse comes to the worse earplugs may give some relief.

SQUINTS

In babies, demand ophthalmic referral whenever mother or doctor suspect their presence. Negative examination does not exclude developing or intermittent squints.

Squints developing for the first time in older children or adults will cause diplopia (relieved by covering the squinting eye). A cause should be diligently sought.

Note: Babies with broad epicanthic folds are as likely to have squints as other babies.

STICKY EYES

Developing within a few days of birth, sticky eyes should be swabbed before being treated with an antibiotic ointment. Recurrence or non-resolution should raise the question of chlamydia infection. Special culture will be required and if positive the baby may be treated with oral erythromycin.

A blocked nasolachrimal duct may contribute to the infection. Mother should be taught how to massage the duct upwards towards the inner canthus so that stasis in the upper blind end is reduced. Patency may well not be achieved until 6–9 months of age and referral for probing should certainly not be before this time.

Note: Reassurance that sticky eyes pose no threat to eyesight helps mother to cope with recurrences.

STYES

Localized infections of the glands of the lid margin. After a few days of painful swelling a bead of pus will be discharged and resolution will take place.

No treatment is necessary though antibiotic ointment may prevent emerging staphylococci from infecting another lash follicle.

Note: Recurrent styes are not a sign of being 'run-down'.

SUNBURN

Fairly common self-inflicted injury. Initial erythema occurs during exposure and disappears shortly afterwards. Delayed erythema, accompanied by pain and discomfort, begins about 3 hours after exposure and persists for about 48 hours. Peeling follows erythema.

Mild cases need use nothing more than a soothing cream four times a day but severer cases may need to take simple analgesics and apply a topical steroid cream for 2–3 days to decrease the inflammatory response.

Note: All cases should avoid further injudicious exposure to sunlight.

'TEETHING'

Occurs supposedly from 6 months to 6 years and may cause some pain, irritability and excess salivation. Although a useful excuse for crying and sleeping difficulties the diagnosis should not be made until general conditions have been excluded.

No treatment is necessary other than paracetamol elixir for pain.

Note: Painful gums may cause hard items of food to be refused.

TENOSYNOVITIS

An inflammatory condition of tendon sheaths which produces pain that is worse during movement of the tendon. Localized tenderness, swelling and crepitus may be present and treatment may be with a short course of a non-steroidal anti-inflammatory drug or more effectively by steroid injection.

Note: This is mostly an isolated condition not associated with systemic disease.

TENNIS ELBOW

Can affect anyone and produces severe pain on the outer side of the arm especially with movements requiring the hand to be turned on its palm. There is localized tenderness over or just below the lateral epicondyle and symptoms will wax and wane until naturally resolving after about 2 years.

A local anaesthetic/steroid injection at the site of maximum tenderness, repeated if necessary one month later, will cure 60 per cent of patients.

Note: Medial epicondylitis is known as golfer's elbow.

THREADWORMS

These live in the bowel in up to 40 per cent of under-10-year-olds. Pruritis ani (particularly nocturnal) is the only symptom that they produce apart from anxiety if an adult worm is seen in the stool. Faecal-oral spread by scratching fingers causes reinfection of the host and new infections in the rest of the family.

As worms live for only 6–8 weeks strict family hygiene for that length of time will resolve the infection. Hygiene advice should be given: affected child should have nails cut short, wear pyjamas and possibly gloves to bed, bathe each morning, carefully washing perianal skin, use own towel, change and wash clothes and bedclothes. In addition all the family should have a strict toilet hygiene. Advice may be coupled with a prescription for a piperazine compound, e.g. Pripsen to be taken in two doses one week apart. Ideally, all members of the family should be treated at the same time, but each should be given an individual prescription.

Note: Prescription without hygiene advice will result in recurrence.

TINNITUS

May be aggravating and distressing. Noises are loudest when the environment is quietest. Wax is the only likely remediable cause as most cases are due to inner ear problems associated with increased age. Most patients are deaf to some degree and their tinnitus will be a persistent problem which no treatment will help.

Note: Other noises can be used to mask out the tinnitus, e.g. keeping a radio on may help a sufferer to get off to sleep.

TOOTHACHE

Usually presents when dentists are not available or feared. If no infection is present then advice about suitable analgesics is all that is necessary. If tooth or gum infection exists then amoxycillin (Amoxil) or erythromycin should be prescribed. In all cases a dental appointment should be advised.

Note: Earache without any other signs of ear disease is often due to pain referred from teeth.

UMBILICAL HERNIA

Varies in size and is common in young babies. Soft and easily reduced with virtually no risk of strangulation. Disappears spontaneously as the baby grows and requires no treatment of any sort.

Note: Parents should understand that the hernia will appear when the baby cries, not that the baby is crying because the hernia has appeared.

UNDESCENDED TESTICLES

Found in 1 in 5 premature and 1 in 25 full-term boys. Most will descend spontaneously by the age of 1 year but if they are not in the scrotum by then orchidopexy is indicated. Operation is probably best carried out between 1 and 2 years and certainly before the age of 5.

Note: A cold surgery or cold hands will activate the cremaster reflex and make examination unreliable.

VARICOSE VEINS

Present, to some degree, in 2 out of 3 adults. Most cases present because of the patient's dissatisfaction with their cosmetic appearance. Aching on standing with heavy, painful and swollen legs may occur as may complications of impaired skin nutrition such as eczema or pigmentation and varicose ulceration.

Diagnosis is straightforward. Clinical localization of incompetent perforating veins is highly inaccurate.

Most cases require no specific treatment. General advice should be given, namely, high roughage diet, keep active, avoiding sitting or standing in the same position for any length of time, avoiding crossing the legs while sitting. Elastic support stockings (full length, standard circular yarn type with no toes) worn regularly will give relief and clinical improvement whether surgical treatment is contemplated or not.

Injection of sclerosing agents is associated with recurrence in 65 per cent of cases after 6 years. With surgery about 25 per cent of patients will need further treatment after 5 years.

Note: Varicose veins are not a contraindication to the pill.

VARICOSE ULCERS

Develop in about 3 per cent of patients with varicose veins especially those with a history of deep vein thrombosis. Ulceration usually occurs in the region of the ankle just above or below the malleoli and may arise spontaneously or after minor injury or infection. Varicose ulcers cause little pain but if present can be relieved by raising the foot.

Treatment is long drawn-out and both the ulcer and the underlying swelling and congestion of the skin need to be dealt with. Raising the leg, with the patient lying flat, followed by compression bandaging is essential for healing. In some cases prolonged bed rest may be needed. A good diet is also essential.

A considerable variety of paste bandages may be used as may Debrisan in resistant cases. Your trainer is likely to have his/her own favourite treatment.

Note: The practice nurse is likely to be more knowledgeable about the management of this condition than you. Do not be afraid to seek his/her advice or refer patients to him/her.

VERRUCAS

These are warts on the feet. Pressure may make them painful on walking. They may be distinguished from simple corns by the presence of blood vessels (paring of the surface of a wart will reveal minute bleeding points).

If they are producing unacceptable pain or deformity, treatment may be indicated. Salicylic acid collodion solution or plasters may be used as may formaldehyde gel (Veracur).

Note: Verrucas are no bar to swimming. If misdirected official bans exist then wearing a waterproof plaster while at the pool will get round them.

WARTS

Generally present for cosmetic reasons because they are only painful if they become secondarily infected or are being traumatized. Before any treatment is undertaken the following factors must be considered: warts naturally resolve (within months in children); there is no drug effective against the wart virus so treatment is empirical; most treatments have poorer results than if the wart is left alone; treatment may be painful while the wart is usually painless; a naturally resolving wart leaves no scars while a badly treated one might; if natural immunity has not developed to the wart virus then a high relapse rate is to be expected.

Most cases need only explanation of the natural history or, if the parents insist on treatment, advice to buy a simple remedy from the chemist and do the work themselves. A few warts causing pain or deformity may need to be removed and if painting with 10 per cent salicylic acid collodion BPC twice daily for 2–3 months does not effect an improvement referral for cautery or cryotherapy may be indicated.

Note: There is no particular reason for doctors to be concerned in the management of this benign lesion and a well-briefed practice nurse should be able to cope with most cases.

WAX IN THE EARS

May accumulate to occlude the meatus and produce deafness, tinnitus or even vertigo. Provided that the ear is not too painful and that there is no suggestion of perforation of the tympanic membrane syringing is the treatment of choice. If wax is hard then the use of olive oil or drops such as Cerumol four times a day for 3 days before syringing will make the task easier. The patient can buy these drops before coming to the nurse or doctor for syringing.

Note: The wax in babies' ears is very soft and may present as a 'runny ear'.

WHOOPING COUGH

Has an incubation period of 7–10 days before the catarrhal phase, which resembles a severe cold, begins. Instead of resolving in 3–4 days fever persists and coughing increases, beginning to occur in bouts and being most prominent at night. After 2 weeks the paroxysmal phase with its characteristic paroxysms followed by vomiting and in many cases whooping, develops and persists for another 3–4 weeks before the child will get better. Infectivity is highest during the catarrhal phase (when the diagnosis is most difficult) and persists for about 4 weeks in all.

No antispasmodic or cough medicine has been shown to affect the cough though an antihistamine, given at night for its sedative effect, may be helpful as, alternatively, might elixir diazepam. A warm humid atmosphere will help relieve coughing spasms and meals are best kept small and frequent if vomiting is troublesome. Although there is little evidence that they help, antibiotics (erythromycin or amoxycillin) are likely to be prescribed at some stage.

Most severe cases tend to occur in children below the age of 6 months and the mainstay of treatment is constant supervision and careful nursing. If paroxysms are severe, social circumstances poor or complications develop then hospital admission is indicated.

Note: Prevention by vaccine is far superior to the largely ineffectual treatment we have to offer established cases.

WRY-NECK

Wry-neck or acute torticollis due to muscular spasm from viral myalgia or secondary to infected cervical glands is slow in onset with a tender muscle found on examination. Treatment consists of rest in a collar, prescription or advice about suitable analgesia and an antibiotic if adenitis is present.

Joint dysfunction causing wry-neck is sudden in onset with severe pain provoked by neck movement. Traction may give quick relief. Stand behind patient who is seated on low stool; put one hand under the chin and the other under the occiput; pull steadily upwards while keeping the neck straight; if pain is worsened *stop*, but, if improved, then repeat several times before putting on collar and giving suitable analgesia.

Note: A cervical collar helps to rest the acutely painful neck and in an emergency can be made by rolling a newspaper to make a flat band wide enough to immobilize the neck when placed round it like a parson's collar and held in place with a scarf.

Chapter 21

Long-term care

Many diseases and disabling conditions cannot be cured and need long-term care.

- Asthma.
- Diabetes.
- Hypertension.
- Epilepsy.
- Thyroid disease.
- Rheumatoid arthritis.
- Chronic bronchitis.
- Heart failure.
- Ischaemic heart disease.

In addition to these, anyone who takes long-term medication should be seen at regular intervals.

OBJECTIVES

- To prevent or delay the progression of chronic disease.
- To prevent or minimize complications of the disease.
- To make the quality of life as good as possible.
- To ensure that the best use is made of available therapies.
- To guard against side effects of medication.
- To ensure that the patient is as self-sufficient and independent as possible.

COMPONENTS OF LONG-TERM CARE

Information

The patient and his/her family need to know as much as possible about:

- The disease and its implications.

- The treatment: how to use it; what to expect from it.
- What help is available and how to obtain it.

Booklets are useful because they can be taken home and read at leisure. Some pharmaceutical companies, special societies and self-help groups provide excellent material. However, 10 to 20 per cent of the population cannot read well enough to understand written explanations of this complexity and even those who can read need personal explanation as well. It is best provided in small amounts and will often have to be repeated on numerous occasions. It is important for those who provide explanations to make sure they are consistent.

Practice organization

It is useful to have an overall plan for caring for patients with long-term problems. Some, such as diabetes, are common enough to consider having a special regular clinic but there will always be some patients who prefer to come at other times. For all patients, some sort of recall system is needed. It is not enough to leave it to the patient to attend for regular follow-up, unless the patient knows as much as the doctor about the possible consequences of inadequate care.

Recall can be organized in various ways: through the appointments system; a simple diary; a card index; disease index; punched cards; or computer. Whatever system is used, it should be needed only if a patient fails to attend, as advised. It therefore involves little administrative time. Follow-up can be linked with repeat prescribing but this fails to identify those who are not taking their drugs and therefore not requesting prescriptions.

The most efficient care results from cooperation within the practice team. Who does what needs to be thought out and will vary depending on the interests and expertise of the personnel available. It is a mistake for doctors to think that they are the only, or even the best, people to perform every task.

Shared care

Many patients with chronic conditions attend hospital outpatient clinics as well as obtaining certain services from their GP. This can lead to an improved standard of care, if there is true cooperation or to an impoverished one, if the areas of responsibility are not clearly understood.

A cooperation card such as is used in antenatal care is a great help and avoids unnecessary letters.

The patients, as well as the doctors, should understand that the hospital element of care is 'as well as' and not 'instead of' the GP part.

Ideally, most care is carried out by the GP and visits to the hospital are for the purpose of advising the GP and not for routine care.

Medication

No one likes taking long-term medication and compliance is variable. To minimize difficulties:

- Make the regimen as simple as possible with few drugs and doses.
- For each drug, ensure the patient understands:
  - what it is for
  - when and how it should be taken
  - what effect to expect
  - what side effects to watch for
  - under what circumstances it should be stopped, the dose changed or the doctor contacted
  - how long it is to be continued
  - whether it is to be taken as well as or instead of other drugs.
- Avoid nonspecific instructions like 'as before', 'as advised' and 'as required'.
- For drugs, such as pressurized inhalers requiring special skills, give someone the task of teaching the skill and of checking from time to time that it is being properly applied.
- Make it simple to obtain repeat prescriptions. There is no reason why someone on long-term treatment should not have three months' supply at a time or postdated prescriptions.

DIABETES

Treatment for diabetes is likely to be initiated in hospital in insulin-dependent diabetics, by the GP for the rest.

Information

Techniques of urine or blood testing and insulin administration are usually taught by nursing staff. It is important for doctors to know what the patient is being taught.

Useful tip: Disposable syringes may be used repeatedly if kept for the same patient. The district nurse is helpful in checking on techniques and giving injections for the blind or disabled.

Understanding. The patient should understand:

- What a hypoglycaemic attack is like, what causes it and what to do both at once and to avoid another.
- The interrelation between diet, activity and insulin dosage.
- What to do if ill.
- When to seek urgent help, e.g. for vomiting.
- The importance of conscientious control.
- Care of the skin and feet.

Information for relatives. It is especially important for the family to know how to recognize the beginning of a hypoglycaemia coma, e.g. by irritability or irrational behaviour, and what to do.

British Diabetic Association. The patient should be given details of the association, which produces some excellent publications and organizes meetings and activities, such as camps for children.

Details of management

A cooperation card or booklet for the patient to carry is extremely useful. One is produced free by Hoechst.

Diet

A diabetic diet should:

- Avoid animal fat.
- Avoid excessive short-acting carbohydrates (sugars).
- Contain plenty of fibre.
- Be balanced with activity, growth and insulin dosage to maintain normal weight.

Food must be eaten regularly in reasonable amounts. Insulin-dependent diabetics usually cooperate well with this but many of the others have a single large meal a day, making control impossible. All diabetics should carry emergency food.

Urine or blood testing

It is better to do random testing occasionally at different times of the day than test sample at same time every day.

Insulin dosage

Dosage should be written down by doctor in booklet or cooperation card and should include type, strength, number of marks on syringe and number of units to be given.

Oral hypoglycaemic agents are of limited value in overweight patients, who should be urged to lose weight.

Activity

Diabetics should be encouraged to lead as normal a life as possible. Food intake may need to be increased or insulin dose reduced if intense or prolonged activity is planned.

Lifestyle

- Regular eating habits are obviously very important.
- Diabetics are at greater risk from smoking than non-diabetics.
- Contraception may pose problems. The pill carries an increased risk in diabetics and the intrauterine contraceptive device is reputed to be less effective than in other women.
- Pregnancy is hazardous to both mother and baby. The diabetes should be well controlled before conception to avoid fetal abnormalities. The woman should discuss this with the consultant before embarking on the pregnancy. Control by frequent blood glucose measurements by patient improves prognosis.

Arrangements for follow-up

Stable diabetic patients without complications may be cared for by their GP alone, but if care is shared with a hospital clinic it should be clearly understood who does what, or important elements of care may be omitted.

Regular routine visits are essential, the frequency depending on the stability and quality of control achieved by the patient.

All diabetics should be seen at least once every six months.

Suggested plan for routine care of diabetes without complications

Every visit (6 months)

Examine interval blood sugar; weight; review patient's tests, well-being, symptoms and ask if there are any queries.

Once a year

Test mid-stream urine specimen, take BP and examine feet. Examination of fundi after short-acting mydriatic.

Every two years

Full central nervous system examination.

HYPERTENSION

Diagnosis

This may be made during screening programme, or at routine examination for hospital admission, employment or life insurance.

Investigation and treatment

In straightforward cases this is normally carried out by the GP; shared care with consultant physician in complicated ones. Most patients will be cared for entirely by the GP.

Before starting treatment:

- Take BP at least three times on different occasions.
- Check: fundi, ECG and chest x-ray, urea and electrolytes, lipoproteins.
- Exclude other causes:
  – coarctation (examine femoral pulses for delay and chest x-ray for rib notching)
  – Conn's syndrome (low serum potassium)

  – Renal disease: examine urine for albumen and microscopically; intravenous pyelogram in the young.
- Refer anyone with papilloedema or if in doubt about diagnosis or about undertaking treatment (very young or very high levels).

Drugs

Introduce stepwise; see frequently until stable.

Non-drug treatment

This is at least as important as drugs. Smoking, weight, exercise, lifestyle.

Information

Leaflets are produced free by some drug companies. Patients need to know

- As much as possible about the disease, its natural history and the importance of treatment.
- The importance of lifestyle and how to cope with stress (e.g. relaxation exercises).
- How to lose weight and stop smoking.
- How to take the drugs.

Details of management

A cooperation card is useful.

Diet

Reduce weight if necessary and then maintain ideal weight. Low animal fats probably sensible, important if lipoproteins abnormal.

Lifestyle

- Stop smoking.
- Recognize stressful factors and avoid or learn to deal with them.
- Practise relaxation – 20 minutes twice a day if possible and when under stress.

- Regular exercise.
- Contraception and pregnancy need care.

Drugs

Dose should be written in cooperation card.

Follow-up

Regular and indefinite (although it may be possible to phase out treatment in some people after a few years).

Arrangements for follow-up

If care is shared with hospital, it should be clearly understood who does what and when. Some sort of recall system is necessary.

Visits have to be frequent at first (e.g. every 2 weeks) until dosage is adjusted to produce desired result. After that, 3-monthly or, in stable cases, 6-monthly visits only may be needed.

Suggested plan for routine care of hypertensives without complications

Can be shared between doctor and nurse.

Every visit

- General inquiry about wellbeing, problems, lifestyle.
- Blood pressure.
- Weight.
- Confirmation of drug regimen.

Every 2 years

- Blood urea and electrolytes.
- Depending on severity: Chest x-ray; ECG; examine fundi.

ASTHMA

Diagnosis

Asthma is often missed as chest clear when patient seen; suspect children with nocturnal cough or coughing and breathlessness after exercise. Useful to be able to exercise patient in or around the surgery.

Information

Success of management depends entirely on how well the patient uses the advice and drugs he is given. The patient needs to:

- Know as much as possible about the disease and its management. Excellent booklets available from Fisons and A&H.
- Recognize trigger factors and avoid them if possible (e.g. household pets) or take sodium cromoglycate before exposure.
- Understand how and when to use drugs – especially the difference between prophylaxis (e.g. sodium cromoglycate) and treatment (e.g. salbutamol).
- Learn technique of using inhaler: pressurized inhalers are frequently misused.
- Lead as normal a life as possible.
- Recognize danger signals when an acute attack fails to respond to treatment.

Relatives need to understand the disease and its management, especially if the patient is a child. A balance must be found between neglect and overcaution.

Details of management

It may be useful for the patient, for short periods, to keep a chart of symptoms and treatment – these are available in the Fisons booklet.

Aims of treatment

- Freedom from wheezing at all times especially at night and on exertion.
- Abolition of acute attacks.

Peak-flow meters

Any one with more than trivial asthma should have a peak-flow meter at home.

Prophylactic treatment

All patients with persistent asthma should be taking prophylactic treatment with sodium cromoglycate or inhaled steroids for basic control. If more than two puffs, twice a day, of inhaled bronchodilator are being used (one inhaler a month), the patient needs regular inhaled steroids. They should be continued when symptoms are controlled. The dose should be increased if an attack is anticipated, e.g. with URTI.

Nebulizers

Bronchodilators and steroids can be given in an electric nebulizer.
  If used in the surgery, beware relapse later.
  Use of home nebulizers should be monitored with a peak-flow meter.
  Spacer devices may be just as good.

Diet

Obesity should be avoided.

Exercise

Regular, protected by sodium cromoglycate if necessary.

Lifestyle

No smoking at all, ever. Emotional stress may be an important trigger factor. May have to avoid polluted atmospheres and allergens (e.g. animals).

Drugs

Aspirin precipitates asthma in some subjects; betablockers should be avoided.

- Have emergency plan for acute attacks; e.g. call doctor, go straight to hospital.
- If a short course of systemic steroids is needed, the daily dose should be written down.
- If the patient has own peak-flow meter, he/she may telephone doctor to report readings.
- Every patient should be observed using an inhaler to check that it is being used correctly.

Arrangements for follow-up

Most symptomatic asthmatics are easy to follow up because they ask for prescriptions. Some, especially children, may have persistent or repeated mild asthma and do not request treatment. Recall system advisable especially for the young.

Frequency depends upon severity, whether seasonal and how much the patient can be relied upon to carry out the treatment correctly.

Suggested plan for routine care of young asthmatic

Every visit (3–6 months)

- General inquiry about wellbeing, exercise tolerance, night wheeze, frequency and severity of symptoms, detailed drug usage. *Note*: watch for those whose activities are limited unnecessarily because of asthma.
- Peak-flow measurement.
- Height and weight.
- Review medication and check that it is being used correctly.

Part Seven
After Training

Chapter 22

The MRCGP examination

WHY TAKE IT?

Membership of the Royal College of General Practitioners (MRCGP) is not a prerequisite for becoming a principal in general practice, yet every year about 2000 trainees take it. Why?

- *An extra qualification*: Many trainees see the examination as a way of enhancing their chances of getting a job at the end of their training.

Although true to an extent since its possession will prove a certain level of attainment, getting a partnership is such a complex business depending on so many factors from the presentation of your application to the suitability of your character, going to all the trouble of taking the MRCGP examination just for this reason is a little excessive.

Possession of membership of the RCGP will certainly influence some prospective partners. Equally it is not unheard of for it to put them off. Nowadays, so many applicants do have it that to be without can leave a trainee feeling very naked.

- *A 'final' examination for the trainee year*: Although the examination is not meant to be a 'final', it can indeed act as a useful gauge to test the success of the previous three years in preparing a trainee for general practice.

Even though not mandatory, it is nice to know that having passed the examination you have reached a certain acceptable level after all your hard work.

- *A key asset for the future.* Although possession of the MRCGP examination is not as yet a necessity in any branch of general practice, there is no certainty that this will always be so. There is every likelihood that at some time possession of an MRCGP examination will be a requirement for becoming a trainer. And there is no knowing how far governmental changes to the family practitioner service may affect rates of pay for those more qualified.

WHAT IS THE MRCGP EXAMINATION?

The MRCGP examination exists to test the performance of candidates who wish to become members of the Royal College of General Practitioners.

It is not a difficult examination (pass rate is around 70 per cent) nor is it designed to act as a hurdle for getting into an exclusive club. It is simply aimed to test the competence of a trainee or practising principal at performing the job for which they have been trained.

The examination is held twice a year, the closing date being about 8 weeks before the start of the written examinations (mid-March for the summer examinations and late August for the winter examinations).

There are three written papers:

- *The multiple choice question paper (MCQ).*
  Sixty stem questions each with five true/false or don't know parts.
  Time: 2 hours.
- *The Modified Essay Question paper (MEQ).*
  Eight or nine questions which each document part of an unfolding story.
  Time: $1\frac{1}{2}$ hours.
- *The Practice Topic Question paper (PTQ).*
  Three questions.
  Time: 2 hours.

These are taken in London or Edinburgh or in a number of regional centres.

There is *one oral* examination, split into two parts, held in London or Edinburgh in the first 2 weeks of July or the second week of December.

All candidates who are invited to attend the orals are sent a logdiary in which they have to keep details of fifty consecutive patients. This is sent to the examiners before the orals and one half of the oral exam is on this. The other oral is a problem-solving oral. Both orals last for between 25 and 30 minutes.

Marking. Each of the three written and two orals carries a total of 20 per cent of the marks.

The pass mark for the written examinations is usually about 50 per cent and all those who get above this level as an average for all three will be invited to attend the orals. Those who are borderline (between about 42 and 50 per cent) will also be asked to attend the orals, thus an invitation to attend the orals does not mean you have passed the written papers section (you are sent no details of your marks after the written papers).

HOW TO DO IT

Everyone has their own techniques for revising and taking examination. It is unwise in the extreme, however, not to do any preparation for this examination.

A guide to the sort of knowledge you should possess can be gained by looking at the broad 'syllabus' of the examination (taken from the book *Future general practitioner—learning and teaching*, and adopted by the college examiners).

Clinical practice: health and disease

The candidate will be required to demonstrate a knowledge of the diagnosis, management and, where appropriate, the prevention of diseases of importance in general practice.

- The range of the normal.
- The patterns of illness.
- The natural history of diseases.
- Prevention.
- Early diagnosis.
- Diagnostic methods and techniques.
- Management and treatment.

Clinical practice: human development

The candidate will be expected to possess a knowledge of human development and be able to demonstrate the value of this knowledge in the diagnosis and management of patients in general practice.

- Genetics.
- Fetal development.
- Physical development in childhood, maturity and ageing.

- Emotional development in childhood, maturity and ageing.
- Intellectual development in childhood, maturity and ageing.
- The range of normal.

Clinical practice: human behaviour

The candidate must demonstrate an understanding of human behaviour particularly as it affects the presentation and management of disease.

- Behaviour presenting to a GP.
- Behaviour in interpersonal relationships.
- Behaviour of the family.
- Behaviour in the doctor–patient relationship.

Medicine and society

The candidate must be familiar with the common sociological and epidemiological concepts and their relevance to medical care and demonstrate a knowledge of the organization of medical and related services in the UK and abroad.

- Sociological aspects of health and illness.
- The uses of epidemiology.
- The organization of medical care in the UK – comparisons with other countries.
- The relationship of medical services to other institutions in society.
- Ethics.
- Historical perspectives of general practice.

The practice

The candidate must demonstrate a knowledge of practice organization and administration and be able critically to discuss recent developments in the evolution of general practice.

- Practice management.
- The team.
- Financial matters.
- Premises.
- Medical records.

- Medicolegal matters.
- Research.

WHAT IT ASSESSES

The examination is designed to assess in a variety of ways the skills of the candidate in:

- Interpersonal communication.
- History taking and information gathering.
- Selecting examinations using investigations and procedures.
- Recording information.
- Interpreting information.
- Problem definition and hypothesis formation.
- Early diagnosis.
- Defining the range of intervention.
- Selecting therapy.
- Providing continuing care.
- Interventive and preventive medicine in relation to: the patient, the family, and the community.
- The organization of his/her practice and himself/herself.
- Teamwork, delegation, and in relating to other colleagues.
- Business methods.
- Communications.

WHAT IS EXPECTED OF THE CANDIDATE

The candidate will be expected to demonstrate appropriate attitudes to his/her patients, colleagues and to the role of the GP. He/she must demonstrate his/her ability to develop and extend his/her knowledge and skills through continuing education.

Absorbing this huge amount of information can be a lengthy process and it is advisable to start revising at least three or four months before the written papers.

TIPS FOR REVISING

- Read widely, especially the *JRCGP* since this obviously reflects the thinking of the college and the subjects that it feels are important. Read also *Update* and the leaders and middle section of the *British Medical Journal* and a selection of the other journals (do not try and read them all but select about half a dozen).

- Read a selection of 'standard works' on general practice (see page 201-202).
- Attend local postgraduate meetings.
- Ask your trainer for regular tutorials aimed at getting you ready for the examination.
- Read the Red Book.
- Make sure you know the constituents of the medicines you use – study the BNF and MIMS.
- Do a few past examinations (available from the college or in books like the *MRCGP Study Book*, A. Moulds, D. Brooks, J. Fry and E. Gambrill, 2nd edition, 1988, Butterworths).
- Attend one of the intensive courses run in many regional hospitals prior to the examination. Do not do this too early since it is of most use after you have revised.

TIPS FOR TAKING THE EXAMINATION
MCQ

- Do not guess.
- Go through the paper answering only those you are certain of, then go back and have a go at those you left blank.
- Answer each question individually – do not get side-tracked by other parts of the same stem question.
- There is a negative marking system (correct answer $+1$, incorrect answer -1; don't know 0).
- There is not an equal distribution of stem questions, e.g.
  - general medicine   12
  - therapeutics   10
  - obs and gynae   6
  - psychiatry   6
  - paediatrics   6
  - ophthalmology   4
  - surgical diagnosis 4
  - ENT   4
  - dermatology   4
  - statistics   2
  - social aspects   2
  - practice organization 2

MEQ

- *Do not* read through the paper before you start.
- Write answers as lists and short notes.
- Do not write about anything other than what is asked.
- This paper tests not only factual recall but the modifying influence of social and cultural factors on both the patient and the doctor – bear this in mind when answering every question.
- $1\frac{1}{2}$ hours is not a lot of time.

PTQ

- Take time before answering the question to think and make notes.
- Answer logically, clearly and do not become too wordy.
- Do not repeat yourself.
- Marks are awarded for presentation, so do not be too messy.
- Purely clinical questions are unlikely.
- Questions usually selected from each of the sections (see above) clinical practice, health and disease, medicine and practice, medicine and society or the practice.
- Questions will often be topical, so keep up to date with what is going on in the papers, the *BMJ* and the *JRCGP*.

Orals

- Arrive so as to give yourself a few minutes to collect your thoughts.
- Do not argue with the examiners, try and make your point logically.
- Try and get in a bit of practice beforehand (ask your trainer to act as an examiner).
- Make sure you know your patients in the log diary. There is nothing to say you cannot take in a list of the patients to jog your memory.
- Do not panic if the examiner picks you up on something or disagrees with you.

USEFUL READING LIST

Common Diseases, Fry J., MTP, 1985 (4th ed.).
Common Sense Use of Medicines, Fry J. *et al.*, MTP, 1988.

Disease Data Book, Fry J. *et al.*, MTP, 1986.

General practice and primary healthcare 1940's-1980's, Nuffield Provincial Hospitals Trust 1988.

MRCGP Study Book, Moulds A. *et al.*, Butterworths, 1988.

Prescribing – What, When & Why? Fry, J., *et al.*, Churchill Livingstone, 1986.

Running a Practice, Jones R. V. H. *et al.*, Croom Helm, 1985 (3rd ed.).

Towards Earlier Diagnosis in Primary Care, Hodgkin K., Churchill Livingstone, 1978 (4th ed.).

Workbook for Trainees in General Practice, Freeling P., John Wright, 1983.

Series for GPs

- Oxford University Press.
- Churchill Livingstone.
- MTP.

All have series of books for GPs and should be consulted.

Chapter 23

Finding your practice

Finding a practice these days is not always an easy matter, so start thinking about what you really want from a practice early, as much as six months before finishing your training.

WHERE TO FIND JOBS

Most jobs are advertised in the *BMJ* although you can also find adverts in the weekly GP newspapers, *GP*, *Pulse*, and *Doctor*.

If you want a single handed practice and you know the area you are interested in then try writing to the local Family Practitioner Committee (FPC) who will send details of any practices that are coming up.

Most practices do advertise, but there are occasions when the availability of a job locally is passed on by word of mouth alone. Ask your trainer, perhaps even your course organizer, and any other local GPs you know to keep their ears open.

Of course if you want to find a job in one of the most popular areas, the rural South West for instance, you may have to move there and content yourself with locums until you strike lucky.

On occasion there may be a vacancy in your training practice. Do not look upon this as a right. The partners are quite at liberty to advertise and interview you like any other candidate. If you do not get the job, however, this can be hurtful.

CHOOSING A PRACTICE

There are more applicants than openings at present. However, it is a mistake to jump at the first job that presents itself. If you have a fair idea of the sort of job you want, then it is well worth waiting until you find it (even if this does mean a bit of hardship). Waiting a year to find the right job is nothing compared to a lifetime working in a place you detest.

Once an advert catches your eye, try to find out a bit about it first, you do not want to waste your (or their) time in applying for something that was not your choice in the first place.

It is best to remember that your ideal practice is probably just that – an ideal. You have to be prepared to make some compromises.

APPLYING FOR A JOB

When sending off an application for a job you need two things: a curriculum vitae (CV); and a covering letter. The principle aim of the exercise is to get yourself noticed – stint at nothing to achieve this goal.

CV

- Presentation is very important. If you cannot produce a good and attractive product on your own then pay someone to do it for you. There are several companies that prepare professional CVs and they advertise in the *BMJ* every week. For around £30 to £40 they send you a questionnaire to fill in about yourself, then return a word-processed copy on nice thick paper.
- Never send photocopies.
- Do not go into detail where it is not needed: it means nothing if you were in the school drama society or were a prefect. The precise subject of your O-levels is also superfluous. Stick to the essentials.
- A good, colour photograph of yourself can be helpful in making your application stand out.
- Present the CV in some form of folder.

Letter

- Many adverts require a hand-written letter. Even if they do not it is best to send one.
- Make sure it is neat, that there are no spelling mistakes and that it is well presented.
- Make it obvious that you are keen and that this is not just another application for you.
- Try making them curious about you; include something that will make them interested to find out more.
- Do not make it too long – it will not be read.

THE INTERVIEW

If you get an interview you are halfway there. But remember, it is you interviewing them almost as much as the other way round.

- Wear something smart.
- Be on time.
- Smile, do not look too tense and nervous. Remember they may be just as worked up as you. Employing a new partner is not something a GP has to do too often.
- Answer all questions truthfully. If there is a skeleton in your closet, or if there is something you think they will not want to hear bring it out in the open – it's bound to happen eventually and if you are honest it can only reflect well upon you.
- Try not to argue, but do not be obsequious. Stand your ground if cornered.
- Always have a few questions ready – try and find out a bit about the practice beforehand.
- Ask about the accounts. This is probably best left to the second interview but it should not be forgotten.
- Do not forget to ask why the vacancy has arisen. It may be that the previous partner decided to leave because of some fundamental problem in the practice. If this is the case then you will probably want to talk.
- Be prepared to bring your spouse (if you have one). It is unfortunate but many practices look upon you as a family unit rather than an individual clinician.

Index

Abdominal pain, 86–7, 135, 136
Abortion, 71
   counselling, 108–9
Access, open, 54–5
Accident and emergency
   department, 52
Acne, 147
Acquired immuno-deficiency
   syndrome (AIDS), 124
Admissions:
   acute, 52
   compulsory, 139–40
Age–sex register, 4, 31–2
Aggressive patients, 131
AIDS (acquired immuno-
   deficiency syndrome), 124
Allergic rashes, 148
Alopecia, 150
Alphafetoprotein screening, 112
Amenorrhoea, 148
Amniocentesis, 112
Antenatal care, 111–3
Anxiety crisis, 138
Appointment systems, 7
Assault, 145
Asthma:
   long-term care, 188–90
   paediatric emergency, 132–3
Athlete's foot, 148
Audits, 4

Back pain, 90–1
Balanitis, 148–9
Baldness, 149
Behaviour, personal, 70

Bell's palsy, 149–50
Bereavement, 139
Birth marks, 150
Blepharitis, 150
'Blue book', 69
Boils, 150
Breast:
   lumps, 87–8
   tenderness, 87–8
British Medical Association
   (BMA), 63
Bumps, 163
Bunions, 151

Car:
   equipment, 125
   trainee allowance, 29
Carpal tunnel syndrome, 152
Catarrh, 151–2
Certificates, issuing, 34–6
Cervical cytology, 113–4
Chest pain, 80–2
Chickenpox, 152
Child guidance clinics, 58
Children:
   colic, 135, 152–3
   cradle cap, 153
   development, 114–5, 116 Fig.
   eczema, 155
   emergencies:
      abdominal pain, 135
      abuse, 128–9
      asthmatic, 132–3
      croup, 131
      crying, 129–31

examination, 128
fever, 130–1
fitting, 133–4
special problems, 128
stridor, 131–2
vomiting and/or diarrhoea,
134–5
enuresis, 155
immunization, 117–9
and eczema, 155
see also individual conditions
Coil (intrauterine contraceptive
device, IUCD), 106–7
Cold sores, 152
Colds, 152
Colic, 3 months or evening, 135,
152–3
Colleagues, relationship with
local, 49
Complaints:
procedure, 71–2
usual reasons, 8, 69
Computerization, medical
records, 32–3
Condom (sheath), 103, 107–8
Confidentiality, 47–8, 71
children, 71
medical records, 33
police and, 57
Confused patients, 131
Conjunctivitis, 153
Consent, patient's, 71
Consultation:
conducting, 6–7
GP/hospital, 6
objectives, 5–6
purposes, 5
Continuous care, 4
records, 31
Contraception, 102–8
combined pill, 103–5

diaphragm and spermicide,
103, 107
intrauterine contraceptive
device (IUCD), coil, 106–7
progestogen only pill (mini-
pill), 105–6
sheath, 103, 107–8
sterilization, 102, 108
Coroner, 56–7
Cough, 82–3
Course organiser, 20
Cradle cap, 153
Cramps, night, 166
Cremation certificates, 36, 56
Croup, 131
Curriculum vitae, 202
Cyst, Meibomian, 163

Dandruff, 153–4
Death, 145–6
certificates, 35–6, 56, 146
diagnosis, 145–6
reporting a, 56–7
unexpected, 146
Defence organizations, 64–5, 69
Deputizing services, 9
misuse of, 70
Diabetes, 182–5
Diaphragm, 103, 107
Diarrhoea, children, 134–5
Disease:
incidence, 4
nature, 4
Disease register, 32
District Health Authorities
(DHAs), 27
Doctor-patient relationship,
47–9
Drug addicts:
notification of, 70
prescribing, 70

Drug companies and representatives, 61
'Drug trials', 61
Drugs:
  prescribing:
    habits, 61
    personal protocol, 75–6
    principles of 75–7
  see also Prescribing
Dysmenorrhoea, 154
Dyspareunia, 96–7
Dysuria and frequency, 88–9

Ear:
  foreign body, 156–7
  otitis externa, 167
  wax, 178
Earache, 154
Eczema, 154–5
Emergencies:
  action, 126–7
  adults, 136–45
    abdominal pain, 136
    alleged assault, 145
    alleged rape, 145
    eyes, 141–4
    psychiatric patients, compulsory admission, 139–40
    psychosocial, 136–9
  death, 145–6
  equipment, 125–6
  home management, 127
  hospital admission, 127
  nature of, 127
  paediatric, see Children, emergencies
  responsibilities, 125
  telephone answering, 126
Employment medical services, 60

Employment outside the practice, 9–10
Enuresis, 155
Epistaxis, 155–6
Examination, 6
Eye:
  acutely painful and/or red, 141–2, 143, 153
  arc, 142
  assessment chart, 143
  conjunctivitis, 141–2, 143, 153
  foreign body, 142, 144, 157
  squints, 172–3
  sticky, 174
  styes, 173

Family planning clinics, 59
Family Practitioner Committees (FPCs), 27, 61
  finance, 28
Family records, 32
Feet, flat, 156, 167
Fever, children, 130–1
Fits, children, 133–4
Fleas, 156
Foreign body:
  in ear, 156–7
  in eye, 142, 144, 157
  in nose, 157

General Medical Council (GMC), 62–3, 69
General Medical Services Committee (GMSC), 63
General practice:
  common complaints about, 16–7
  compared to hospital practice, 3–4
  reasons for choosing, 15–6
  special features, 3–4

types of, 11–2
General practitioner:
  assistant, 43
  as employer, 42–4
  principals:
    number in UK, 11
    number of women, 12
  as trainer, 20, 22–3, 44
Glandular fever, 157–8
Grief, 139
Group practice, 11

Halitosis, 158
Hayfever, 158–9
Headache, 78–80
Health centres, 11, 42
Health visitors, 38
Hernia, umbilical, 175–6
History, 6
Home visits, 7–8
Hospital services, 52–5
Hyperhidrosis, 159
Hypertension, 185–7
Hyperventilation, 99–100

Imaging department, open
  access, 54–5
Immunization:
  child:
    administration, 118
    contraindications, 118
    eczema, 155
    whooping cough:
      contraindications, 117
      discussion with parents,
        115–7
    travel, 121, 122
Impetigo, 159–60
Indigestion, 84–6
Influenza, 160
Insect bites and stings, 160–1

Insomnia, 100–1, 161
Insurance reports, 35, 50–1
  examination, 51
Interview expenses, 29
In toeing, 161–2
Intrauterine contraceptive
  device (IUCD) or coil, 106–7

Joint Committee on Postgraduate Training in General
  Practice (JCPTGP), 19
  certificate of vocational
    training, 18–9

Knees, knock, 162

Laryngitis, 162
Lice, 162–3
Local Medical Committee
  (LMC), 64
Local services, 56–60
Locums, 44
Long-term care:
  components of, 180–2
  conditions requiring, 180
  medication, 182
  objectives, 180
  practice organization, 181
  shared, 181–2
    cooperation card, 183
  see also individual conditions
Lumps, 163

Malaria prophylaxis:
  drugs, 122
  general measures, 122
Marriage guidance, 59
Maternity certificates, 35
Maternity leave, as GP trainee,
  29
Measles, 163

Medical checkups, 120
Medical records, 30–3
  A4 size, 32
  computerized, 32–3
  confidentiality, 33
  staff access, 33
Medical register, 62, 69
Medical reports, 35
Melanoma, malignant, 164
Menopause, 164
Metatarsus varus, 161–2
Midwives, 39
Moles, 164
Mouth ulcers, 164–5
MRCGP examination:
  aims of, 197
  pass mark, 195
  reading list, 199–200
  reasons for taking, 193–4
  revision tips, 197–8
  sitting, tips, 198–9
  structure, 194–5
  syllabus, 195–7
Mumps, 165

Nappy rash, 165–6
Neck pain, 91–3
NHS certificates, 34–5
Nose:
  foreign body, 157
  polyps, 166
Nurses:
  district, 38
  practice, 40–1
    training, 41
  specialized, 39

Obesity, 167
Otitis externa, 167
Out of hours cover, 9, see also
  Deputizing services

Out-toeing, 167
Overseas travel advice:
  general advice, 120–1
  immunization, 121, 122
  see also Malaria prophylaxis

Pain:
  abdominal, 86–7, 135, 136
  back, 90–1
  chest, 80–2
  neck, 91–3
Palpitations, 97–9
Panic crisis, 138
Partners, relationships with, 49
Partnership:
  characteristics of good, 43
  contracts, 43
Pathology department, open
  access, 54–5
Patient management, principles
  of, 75
Pertussis (whooping cough)
  vaccination, 117–19
Piles, 167–8
Pill:
  combined, 103–5
  progestogen only (mini),
    105–6
Pityriasis rosea, 168
Police, 57
Police surgeons, 57
Polyps, nasal, 166
Postgraduate adviser, 19
Practice agreement, 43
Practice finance, allowances, 43
Practice finding your, 43, 201–3
  advertisements, 201
  application, 202–3
  choosing a practice, 201–3
  curriculum vitae, 202
  interview, 203

Practice lists, size, 4, 11–12
Practice manager, 40
Practice staff, emergencies, 125
Practice team:
    advantages/disadvantages, 37
    composition, 37
    health authority staff, 37–9
    inappropriate delegation, 70
    relationship with, 50
    staff employed by GP, 39–41
    see also individual members
Preconception counselling,
    109–11
Pregnancy, termination, *see*
    Abortion
Pregnancy advice centres, 59
Premenstrual syndrome (PMT),
    168–9
Prescribing:
    abuse of privileges, 70
    repeat, 8–9
    unseen patient, 8–9
Prescription cards, personal,
    9, 31
Presentation, 3
Private certificates, 35
Private practice, 50
Professional conduct, 62–3
Psoriasis, 169
Psychiatric patients, compulsory
    admission, 139–40
Psychosocial emergencies, 136–
    9
Psychotic, acutely, 131–2

Rape, alleged, 145
Rashes, allergic, 148
Raynaud's disease, 169
Receptionists, 39–40
Referrals, 49, 52–4

Regional Health Authorities,
    27–8
Regional medical officers
    (RMOs), 60–1
Registrar of births and
    deaths, 56
Removal expenses, as
    trainee, 28
Remuneration, as trainee, 28–9
Rent, excess, as trainee, 29
Repeat prescribing, records, 31
Research registers, 31
Research studies, opportunity
    for, 4
Ringworm, 170
Royal College of General
    Practitioners (RCGP), 64
    membership examination, *see*
        MRCGP examination
Royal Society of Medicine
    (RSM), 65
Rubella, 170

Salary, as trainee, 28
Scabies, 171
School health services, 57–8
Screening, private sector, 60
Second opinions, 53–4, 123–4
Secretaries, 39
Sex therapy, 59
Sheath (condom), 103, 107–8
Shingles, 171
Sick doctors:
    GMSC health committee, 63
    National Counselling Service
        for, 63
Sick leave, trainee, 29
Sickness certificates, 34
Single-handed practice, 11
Sinusitis, 171–2
Snoring, 172

Social services, 39, 58–9
Soiling, 172
Sore throats, 172
Spermicides, 107
Squints, 172–3
Sterilization, 102, 108
Stridor, 131–2
Styes, 173
Suicide threats/attempts, 138
Sunburn, 173–4

Teething, 174
Telephone:
  costs as trainee, 29
  using the, 8
Tennis elbow, 174
Tenosynovitis, 174
Terminal care, 124
Testicles, undescended, 176
Threadworms, 174–5
Tinnitus, 175
Toenails, ingrowing, 160
Toothache, 175
Torticollis, acute, 179
Trainer, 20, 22–3, 44
Treatment, 6
  principles of, 75–7

Ulcers, mouth, 164–5
Urticaria, 148
Vagina:
  abnormal bleeding, 94–6
  discharge, irritation, 93–4
Varicose ulcers, 176–7
Varicose veins, 176
Vasectomy, 102, 108

Verrucas, 177
Vertigo, acute, 140–1
Violent patients, 131
Vision, sudden loss of, 144–5
Visiting bag, equipment, 125
Vocational training, 18–9
  contracts, 23
  DIY schemes, 21
  formal schemes, 20
  guidelines, 21–3
  JCPTGP certificate, 18–9
  pay, conditions, 23–4, 28–9
  problems, 23–4
  selecting a practice, 22
Voluntary services, 59–60
Vomiting, children, 134–5

Warts, 177–8
Whooping cough (pertussis),
  178–9
  vaccination, 115–7
Work, off-duty, as trainee, 29
Wry-neck (acute torticollis), 179